The Peptide Book

CRAFTED BY SKRIUWER

Copyright © 2024 by Skriuwer.

All rights reserved. No part of this book may be used or reproduced in any form whatsoever without written permission except in the case of brief quotations in critical articles or reviews.

At **Skriuwer**, we're more than just a team—we're a global community of people who love books. In Frisian, "Skriuwer" means "writer," and that's at the heart of what we do: creating and sharing books with readers worldwide. Wherever you are in the world, **Skriuwer** is here to inspire learning.

Frisian is one of the oldest languages in Europe, closely related to English and Dutch, and is spoken by about **500,000 people** in the province of **Friesland** (Fryslân), located in the northern Netherlands. It's the second official language of the Netherlands, but like many minority languages, Frisian faces the challenge of survival in a modern, globalized world.

We're using the money we earn to promote the Frisian language.

For more information, contact : **kontakt@skriuwer.com** (www.skriuwer.com)

TABLE OF CONTENTS

CHAPTER 1: INTRODUCTION TO PEPTIDES

- Basic definition and importance of amino acids
- Early discoveries and modern research techniques
- Comparison with larger proteins
- Widespread presence and fundamental roles in the body

CHAPTER 2: THE BASICS OF PEPTIDE STRUCTURE

- Formation of peptide bonds and amino acid sequences
- Primary, secondary, and tertiary structures
- Differences between short peptides and long proteins
- Significance of shape and folding on function

CHAPTER 3: PEPTIDES AND THEIR ROLE IN THE BODY

- Cell-to-cell communication and signaling
- Influence on hormones and metabolic processes
- Importance in immune support and tissue repair
- Links to brain function and nerve activity

CHAPTER 4: PROTEINS VS. PEPTIDES

- Key distinctions in size and complexity
- Unique structural features and folding patterns
- Different roles in biological processes
- Comparisons in stability and delivery methods

CHAPTER 5: THERAPEUTIC USES OF PEPTIDES

- Peptide-based drugs for various health conditions
- Benefits in hormone regulation, wound healing, and more
- Challenges in stability and targeted delivery
- Examples of approved peptide medications

CHAPTER 6: PEPTIDES IN SKIN CARE

- Reasons for including peptides in topical products
- Types of peptides used for firmness, hydration, or soothing
- Effect of concentration and stability on results
- Combining peptides with other skincare ingredients

CHAPTER 7: PEPTIDES AND SIGNS OF AGING

- Collagen and elastin support through peptide signals
- Role of peptides in muscle tone and connective tissue
- Impact on immune and metabolic changes in aging
- Balancing realistic expectations with peptide potential

CHAPTER 8: PEPTIDES FOR HAIR AND NAIL HEALTH

- How keratin structures relate to peptide activity
- Scalp environment and nail matrix support
- Popular peptides in shampoos, conditioners, and treatments
- Importance of diet and overall care alongside peptides

CHAPTER 9: PEPTIDES AND WEIGHT MANAGEMENT

- Peptide hormones that regulate hunger and fullness
- Effects on blood sugar and metabolic balance
- Combining peptides with nutrition and exercise strategies
- Safety considerations and realistic timelines

CHAPTER 10: PEPTIDES IN ATHLETIC PERFORMANCE

- Recovery support through peptide signaling
- Potential for muscle growth and endurance
- Ethical and regulatory concerns in sports
- Balancing training regimens with safe peptide use

CHAPTER 11: REGULATIONS AND SAFETY GUIDELINES

- Roles of government agencies in peptide oversight
- Quality standards (GMP) and labeling rules
- Dealing with counterfeit or unapproved products
- Global differences in regulation and enforcement

CHAPTER 12: RESEARCH AND CLINICAL TRIALS

- Stages of peptide discovery and testing
- Lab, animal, and human trial processes
- Common challenges in stability and efficacy
- Future directions with personalized and accelerated research

CHAPTER 13: PEPTIDES AND MENTAL HEALTH

- Neuropeptides involved in mood and stress responses
- Links to anxiety, depression, and social behavior
- Potential therapies and ongoing clinical studies
- Challenges in blood-brain barrier delivery

CHAPTER 14: PEPTIDE MANUFACTURING AND INDUSTRY PRACTICES

- Chemical synthesis (solid-phase and liquid-phase)
- Purification, quality control, and GMP standards
- Scaling up for pharmaceuticals and cosmetics
- Emerging greener, more efficient production methods

CHAPTER 15: MISCONCEPTIONS ABOUT PEPTIDES

- Clarifying myths like "all peptides are the same"
- Understanding realistic timelines for change
- Differences between natural and synthetic sources
- Recognizing hype vs. evidence-based claims

CHAPTER 16: NATURAL SOURCES OF PEPTIDES

- Peptides in daily foods and fermented products
- Marine and plant-derived defensive peptides
- Influence of cooking and processing on peptide content
- Ethical and sustainable collection from nature

CHAPTER 17: FUTURE PROSPECTS IN PEPTIDE SCIENCE

- Advances in personalized therapies and vaccine design
- Smart delivery systems, AI-based peptide discovery
- Potential for environmental and agricultural solutions
- Balancing innovation, cost, and ethical concerns

CHAPTER 18: ETHICS OF PEPTIDE USE

- Medical vs. enhancement purposes
- Fairness in sports and social equity
- Transparency, informed consent, and regulation
- Handling cultural, environmental, and moral issues

CHAPTER 19: COMBINING PEPTIDES WITH OTHER APPROACHES

- Synergy with diet, exercise, and healthy lifestyles
- Integration with existing medical treatments
- Mind-body techniques for mental and physical gains
- Adjusting dosage or routines for sustainable results

CHAPTER 20: CREATING A PERSONAL PEPTIDE PLAN

- Defining goals and checking health baselines
- Selecting reliable peptides and product forms
- Building a supportive daily schedule
- Monitoring progress, adapting, and maintaining results

Chapter 1: Introduction to Peptides

Peptides are tiny chains made up of building blocks called amino acids. These building blocks come together in specific sequences. Their shapes and lengths vary, but they are smaller than proteins. When we look at proteins, we see a much larger structure with many amino acids. Peptides, on the other hand, are often formed by fewer amino acids. Yet, despite their smaller size, peptides are very important in many parts of the body.

Amino acids are sometimes called the "letters" of proteins and peptides. Each amino acid is like a small unit. When they join, they create long or short chains. The body has many ways to use these chains. Some are used to help cells talk to each other, so signals can be passed from one place to another. Others help with growth, repair, or keeping the body safe from harm.

There are also natural peptides found in different parts of nature. Plants, animals, and even small life forms like bacteria can produce peptides. For example, certain insects have peptide-based chemicals that fight off things that could harm them. Some plants also make peptides that keep them safe from hungry pests. Even germs use peptides in different ways, such as sending signals to form protective layers. The wide presence of peptides in nature shows how powerful and flexible they can be. Over time, humans have learned to study and use them for many reasons.

One of the earliest peptide-related findings in science came when researchers noticed that certain extracts from plants or tissues had special effects. They did not know what these extracts were made of at first, but they saw that small amounts could cause big changes in the body. Scientists were amazed by how active these substances could be. As tools improved, they found that many of these extracts contained peptides. This led people to pay attention to these small chains and figure out how to isolate and study them.

In modern times, peptides have become much easier to research. Advanced machines and techniques let scientists see their structure and figure out their functions. Researchers use tools like mass spectrometry to identify peptides in samples. They also grow them in labs by combining amino acids in the right order. When they do this, they can create peptides that might not exist naturally.

This gives them a chance to test new possibilities and see if they can help people.

Because of these efforts, a branch of science and medicine focuses on how peptides can be used to solve problems. We now know of many ways that peptides affect our bodies. Some peptides control how cells talk to each other. Others work in the immune system to protect us. Some peptides can affect how hungry or full we feel. They can also affect our mood and reactions to stress. The long list of peptide functions has led to a greater appreciation of what these small chains can do.

As researchers learned more, they found that some peptides help cells grow or heal. This property has drawn attention from people who want to use these peptides to help repair tissue or speed up healing from wounds. Doctors and scientists look for ways to guide these natural processes in a useful way. For example, there are peptides that might help new blood vessels form. This can be very helpful for tissues that need better blood flow, such as injured skin or muscle.

Peptides also play a role in how the body handles sugar and other energy sources. Some peptides help regulate insulin, which helps the body manage sugar in the blood. When we have too much sugar in the blood, it can harm organs. Proper management helps keep us healthy. This is a major topic for people who study diabetes and other metabolic issues. They want to see if peptides can be made into treatments.

The fact that peptides are smaller than proteins has some benefits when developing treatments. Smaller molecules can sometimes enter tissues or cells more easily. This can make them useful for targeting specific areas in the body. Also, peptides can be more stable and less likely to cause unwanted reactions, compared to certain larger proteins. Of course, every substance in the body can have side effects, so it is important for researchers to test each peptide carefully.

Beyond medical uses, peptides have also become popular in the beauty industry. Many skin creams now have peptides that are said to help the skin look and feel healthier. The idea is that these peptides can support the building blocks of the skin, like collagen and elastin. Collagen is important for skin structure, and elastin helps the skin stay flexible. Over time, the levels of these proteins can drop, which can cause changes in how skin looks. People hope that peptides in creams or lotions might help the skin stay in better shape. We will look at this more in later chapters, but it is one example of how peptides are found in everyday items.

Peptides also show up in health supplements. You might see them mentioned on product labels. Some supplements aim to help with muscle growth, repair, or other body processes. While some people believe strongly in these products, it is important to check reliable sources and talk to experts before starting any new supplement. Scientists continue to investigate how well certain peptide-based supplements work and whether they are safe in the long run.

In some cases, the body makes fewer peptides as we grow older. This may have effects on how well our body recovers, how our immune system functions, and other processes. Researchers are studying ways to replace or support these reduced peptides. They wonder if giving the body more of the peptides it loses over time could improve well-being. This is not fully understood yet, so experts must continue testing to see if it works as hoped.

One challenge is that peptides can sometimes be broken down quickly in the body. Enzymes that break down proteins can also break down peptides, especially if the peptide is small or fragile. Scientists look for ways to protect peptides so they can last long enough to do their job. This might involve changing the structure of the peptide or putting it into a special delivery system, like a capsule or an injection that helps it survive in the bloodstream.

Another point to think about is how specific peptides are. Some peptides might have a strong effect on one function in the body, but also cause side effects somewhere else. Because of this, researchers must run many tests to see how each peptide behaves under different conditions. They test different doses and formulas to find a balance between effectiveness and safety. Medicines must be tested in small steps, moving from lab studies to controlled trials with volunteers, before they are widely used.

Throughout history, humans have looked for substances that can support health. Peptides are just one of the many things we have discovered. They are not new, because nature has used them for millions of years. But our ability to understand them and make them has grown a lot in recent decades. This has led to new treatments for some illnesses, as well as new ways to care for skin and hair. It has also sparked interest in using peptides for sports performance, weight balance, and more.

One reason peptides have gained attention is that they can be designed to target very specific goals. For instance, if scientists know that a certain receptor on a cell is involved in a disease, they can try to build a peptide that fits that receptor. This is somewhat like making a key that fits a certain lock. The lock is the receptor, and the key is the peptide. If they match, the peptide can activate or block that receptor. This might help treat the condition by shutting down harmful actions or enhancing helpful ones.

There are also peptides that come from everyday foods. For example, some peptides are made when certain types of proteins in food are broken down. The gut can absorb these small peptides. Researchers are still investigating how these dietary peptides affect health and whether they have benefits, like lowering blood pressure or helping with digestion. Some studies suggest that certain peptides from milk, soy, or fish might be helpful, but this area of research is still growing.

It is important to remember that not all peptides are safe for everyone. Some might cause allergies or other issues. Also, not all peptides are legal to buy or use. In some places, peptides used for performance may be regulated or restricted. That is why knowing the rules and regulations is helpful. In a later chapter, we will talk more about these policies and how they affect people who want to use peptides for different reasons.

While this first chapter offers an overall look at peptides, each upcoming chapter will focus on a more specific area. We will talk about how peptides are built, the difference between peptides and proteins, and the many ways they can help in health and beauty. We will also discuss research in this field, current uses, safety points, and future possibilities. This book aims to share clear information and offer a deeper understanding of peptides. By knowing the basics, you can appreciate why these tiny chains are so important in many fields.

In the past, people may have only heard the word peptide in science textbooks or advanced health articles. But the topic is no longer limited to labs. Peptides are part of everyday discussions in medical news, beauty tips, and even athletic circles. Some sports people look into peptides for muscle and recovery. Others ask about them for weight management or for support in the aging process.

Because of all this, peptides have become a topic of great interest, and it can be confusing to figure out all the details. That is why it helps to have a clear explanation, so you can make sense of these small but powerful chains.

In medicine, peptides serve as treatments in some areas. A good example is the group of peptide drugs that help with certain hormonal issues or autoimmune conditions. While not all these drugs are widespread, those that have been approved can make a big difference for patients. They can fill in the gap where the body does not make enough of a needed peptide or help fix imbalances.

In addition, some people hope that peptides might help with problems like damage to cartilage or other body tissues that do not heal easily. The body does have ways to repair these tissues, but sometimes the process is slow. Researchers think certain peptides might speed this up by signaling the cells involved in repair. These signals might be turned up or guided by the presence of the right peptide.

Peptides are also a topic in the field of healthy living. People read about them and wonder if adding them to their diet or using them in creams or supplements can help them stay fit. While there are claims of various benefits, it is wise to look for real scientific data. Not every product that lists "peptides" will have proven effects. This does not mean peptides do not work. It just means that some products might not have enough of the right type of peptide, or they might not have the right delivery method.

It is clear that peptides can do much in the body, but there is still a lot to learn. The study of peptides is ongoing. New discoveries appear every year. For instance, scientists might find a new peptide in a plant, discover how it works, and then see if it has applications in human health. They might even change the peptide slightly to make it more stable or more effective. Over time, these steps can lead to new treatments or products.

For now, it is good to approach peptides with both interest and care. They hold potential in health, beauty, and many other fields, but it is important to rely on proper research and credible sources before using any new peptide-based approach. This book will give details and examples so that the idea of peptides is not mysterious. Instead, you will be able to see why scientists are so interested in these chains of amino acids and how they may be used in everyday life.

In the next chapters, we will talk about the basics of peptide structure, compare them with proteins, and explore the many ways they work in the body. By keeping an open mind and looking at the data, you can form your own opinion on the role of peptides. Some people find that certain peptide-based products or treatments are helpful for them. Others may not need or benefit from them, depending on their goals and body chemistry. With the right information, you can decide what is useful in your own life.

Many experts see peptides as one of the important areas of science to watch. They believe that as we understand more about them, we may find better ways to address health concerns. At the same time, it is wise to remember that peptides are not magical. They are biological tools that work under specific conditions. The best path is to mix them with other healthy habits, like balanced eating and physical activity, for those who want to use them. In chapters ahead, we will go over specific topics, such as skin care peptides, hair care peptides, and how the body's natural peptide levels change over time.

The world of peptides is vast, but it does not have to be overwhelming. It starts with a simple concept: small chains of amino acids can do big things. By grasping that basic idea, you have taken the first step in understanding peptides on a deeper level. And now that we have set the stage, we can examine the core details of how these chains form, work, and compare with other substances in the body.

Chapter 2: The Basics of Peptide Structure

Peptides are made of amino acids joined together by bonds known as peptide bonds. A peptide bond links the end of one amino acid to the beginning of the next. When two amino acids bond, we call it a dipeptide. If there are three, it is a tripeptide, and so on. The length of the chain can vary greatly. Some peptides have just two or three amino acids. Others might have dozens. If the chain gets very long, it is usually called a protein. The line between a long peptide and a protein is not always strict, but often peptides are seen as having fewer than 50 amino acids.

To understand peptide structure, let us look at the amino acids themselves. Each amino acid has two special groups. On one side, it has an amino group (often with nitrogen), and on the other side, it has a carboxyl group (with carbon and oxygen). When a peptide bond forms, the carboxyl group of one amino acid joins with the amino group of the next, releasing a molecule of water in the process. This reaction is known as a condensation reaction.

The specific order of amino acids in a peptide is called its primary structure. Each amino acid is often shown by a letter or three-letter code. For example, glycine is "Gly," and alanine is "Ala." When scientists write the sequence, they line up letters or codes. This is important because the order of amino acids decides the shape and the function of the peptide. Even changing one amino acid can make a big difference.

Once the peptide has a sequence, it may fold into a shape. With small peptides, the shape is often simple, but sometimes it can form loops or other structures. Larger peptides might have areas called alpha helices or beta sheets, which are more organized patterns. These patterns are more common in bigger chains, like proteins, but some peptides also form them. Each shape is stabilized by different interactions in the chain, such as hydrogen bonds.

The body uses enzymes to help make or break down peptide bonds. For instance, when you eat protein, enzymes in your stomach and intestines cut the proteins into smaller peptides and amino acids. These smaller pieces can then be absorbed into the bloodstream. Once inside the body, they can be used to build new peptides or proteins as needed. The body is clever at handling these materials to support growth, repair, and maintenance.

Because peptides can be made by the body or found in foods, people may wonder how a lab-made peptide fits into the picture. In research settings, scientists often synthesize peptides by piecing amino acids together in an exact order. This can be done with machines that automate the process. Synthetic peptides can be tested to see if they have certain properties, such as the ability to bind to specific receptors or signals. This helps researchers create medicines or treatments for certain conditions.

One example is a well-known synthetic peptide that helps with blood sugar control. Scientists managed to copy a peptide found in nature and improve it, making it more stable in the bloodstream. This is important because natural peptides can be broken down quickly. By changing a few amino acids or modifying them slightly, they can last longer in the body. This technique is very useful for drug development.

Another aspect of peptide structure is the presence of side chains. Each amino acid has a side chain that can be different, like a small group of atoms for glycine or a more complex group for tryptophan. These side chains can be charged or neutral, and some can be hydrophobic (water-hating) or hydrophilic (water-loving). When the peptide folds, these side chains can interact with each other and with water. These interactions shape how the peptide behaves.

Some peptides exist in rings rather than straight chains. These are called cyclic peptides. The ends of the chain can connect, or some side chains can form bonds to make loops. This looping can protect the peptide from being broken down by enzymes in the body. Certain antibacterial peptides found in nature are cyclic. They can insert themselves into harmful cells and create holes or disrupt processes, helping organisms defend against infections.

The concept of peptide structure also includes the idea of modifications. A peptide can have sugars or other chemical groups added. These decorations can change how the peptide folds or how it interacts with receptors. Sometimes, a phosphate group is added, turning the peptide on or off in signaling pathways. The cell uses enzymes to make these changes when needed. This process is often well-regulated, allowing the cell to control the function of peptides and proteins.

When we talk about the basics of peptide structure, we also need to look at how structure connects to function. Because peptides are smaller than proteins, they can move into areas that big proteins cannot. This can be beneficial if you want to get a molecule to pass through the skin or reach a part of the body blocked by certain barriers. Yet, being small can also be a downside. Small peptides may degrade faster. That is why many researchers pay attention to stabilizing peptides without losing their function.

Peptides can also act as signals between cells. For instance, in the body, there are peptide hormones that move through the bloodstream and tell distant cells what to do. An example is insulin, which is made up of chains of amino acids. It helps cells take in sugar from the blood. Though insulin is often seen as a protein because it is a bit longer, it still shows how these amino-acid chains can regulate large-scale functions. Other peptide hormones control things like growth, stress response, and appetite.

Some peptides specialize in linking together to form bigger structures. Collagen, found in skin and connective tissue, is made of three chains twisting around one another. This triple helix shape gives collagen strength. Though collagen is often called a protein, it is interesting to note that it is made up of repeating peptide units. This helps illustrate the idea that the line between peptide and protein can sometimes blur. It depends on length and complexity, but both are built from the same basic blocks.

For people new to the subject, the main takeaway is that every peptide starts with a specific sequence of amino acids. This sequence is key to what it does. If someone knows the sequence, they can guess the shape, and from there, they can guess how it might function. Of course, in reality, the path from sequence to function can be tricky. Many lab experiments are needed to confirm how a peptide will act in a real biological system.

Learning about peptide structure also includes understanding how fragile these chains can be. Heat, strong acids, or strong bases can break peptide bonds. That is why cooking can change the texture of food by unraveling proteins and cutting them into peptides. In the body, enzymes do something similar, though in a more controlled and precise way. This breakdown process is crucial for digestion, recycling of old proteins, and energy production.

Because of these properties, certain methods are used to deliver peptide-based medicines. Injections are common, since swallowing a peptide pill might lead to the peptide breaking apart in the stomach. Researchers look for ways to protect peptide drugs from acids and enzymes in the digestive system. Special coatings or formulations might help. In some cases, nasal sprays or patches are tested as alternative ways to get peptides into the bloodstream.

In the scientific community, there is a lot of interest in designing peptides that can bind to harmful molecules in the body and help remove them. This is somewhat like giving the body little "sponges" that soak up the harmful targets. Alternatively, peptides can be attached to tiny carriers, like nanoparticles, to deliver them to specific cells, such as tumor cells. These approaches involve careful planning of the peptide structure, so it will stick to the right targets but remain stable long enough to do its job.

Different fields find different uses for peptides. In agriculture, some researchers try to design peptides that protect crops from pests. These might be sprayed on plants or engineered into the plant's own system. In veterinary science, peptides might help animals fight infections without relying solely on antibiotics. Each field has its own reasons to explore these small chains.

In day-to-day life, peptides show up in various items we might see at the store. Shampoos, conditioners, face creams, and serums may list peptides in the ingredient list. These peptides might aim to help strengthen hair or help skin stay moisturized. While the exact science behind each product can vary, the reason they are included is usually because peptides can signal or support certain tissues. The peptides in these items are often synthetic versions of natural peptides or fragments of proteins.

Another interesting part of peptide structure is how it can be recognized by cell receptors. These receptors are often on the surface of cells. A cell might have thousands of receptors that recognize different signals. If a peptide has the right shape, it can fit into a receptor like a puzzle piece. This can tell the cell to start or stop a process. For example, if the peptide signals muscle growth, then attaching to the receptor might tell muscle cells to grow larger or repair. If the peptide signals the release of enzymes, then the cell might start producing those enzymes.

Since peptides are so specific, researchers sometimes aim to make them even more selective. They might remove parts of the sequence that cause side effects. Or they might add certain chemical groups that only fit into the receptor in one tissue. The end goal is to create a substance that gives benefits while minimizing harm. This is part of the bigger field of drug design and development.

In summary, the structure of peptides comes down to amino acids, peptide bonds, and the shapes that form as a result of interactions. Their small size and adaptability allow them to be used by living organisms for many tasks. Whether we are talking about signaling, defense, or building materials, peptides fill key roles. Understanding the basics of peptide structure helps us appreciate why they can have so many uses in health, beauty, and research.

As you think about how peptides work at this structural level, remember that each peptide is unique. The slightest change in sequence or shape can make it do something entirely different. This is why the variety of natural peptides is so large. Over countless generations, organisms evolved many types of peptides for different functions. Now, humans are learning to harness this variety, both by studying nature and by designing our own synthetic peptides.

In the next chapters, we will see how peptides compare with proteins in greater detail and how they function in the body. We will also explore the many ways they can be used for health and the reasons why they have become popular in the field of beauty. But before moving on, it is worth remembering that it all begins with this basic structural principle: a chain of amino acids joined by peptide bonds. From this simple foundation, an entire realm of possibilities opens up.

Keeping the structure of peptides in mind also helps when evaluating products or news about new peptide discoveries. If someone claims that a certain peptide can pass through the stomach and do specific tasks without being broken down, it is important to see if there is data to show it. Sometimes, a product might need a special protective method, because the structure of peptides is such that they can be broken down in the gut. By understanding these basics, you can ask better questions and get more accurate answers.

The science around peptide structure will continue to advance. New tools allow scientists to design peptides with precise shapes. In the future, we might see more targeted peptide therapies for specific illnesses, with fewer side effects than older treatments. We might also see broader uses for peptides in everyday goods. No matter how they are used, though, the core idea remains: small amino acid chains with a specific sequence can have strong and targeted effects on biological systems.

As we proceed in this book, you will learn more about how peptides and proteins differ, the diverse roles of peptides in the body, and the ways they are applied in clinical settings. We will also talk about how they help skin, hair, and other tissues. By keeping in mind the basic structure described here, you will be ready to understand more advanced details. Every topic will build on what we have covered so far, so the foundation of amino acids and peptide bonds is an important starting point.

Chapter 3: Peptides and Their Role in the Body

Peptides are short chains of amino acids that work in many ways to support normal life processes. They can send signals between cells, help the body fight off infections, and even support repair of tissues. In this chapter, we will explore these roles in detail and look at how peptides help different organs and systems work properly.

---

1. Cell-to-Cell Communication
A key part of how the body stays healthy involves cells sending messages to one another. Cells use different kinds of signaling molecules to do this, and peptides are among the most important. A cell might release a small peptide, which travels to a neighboring cell. That next cell has receptors on its surface. If the shape of the peptide matches one of these receptors, the receptor will sense the peptide and cause changes inside the cell. These changes can include turning certain genes on or off, causing the cell to produce certain substances, or making it grow, shrink, or adjust in other ways.

Because peptides are smaller than large proteins, it can be easier for them to travel in certain parts of the body. They may pass through thin membranes or navigate tight spaces that bigger molecules cannot. This can be helpful when signals need to reach cells in distant areas. Many peptide messengers work best over short distances, but some can move through the bloodstream. The shape of each peptide matters a lot. If the shape does not match the receptor, the cell will not respond.

---

2. Hormones and Regulation
While some hormones are large proteins or steroids, others are short peptide hormones. These include substances that help control hunger, thirst, growth, and more. One well-known example is ghrelin, often called the "hunger hormone." Ghrelin is a peptide that is released in the stomach. When your stomach is empty, ghrelin levels rise and signal the brain that you are hungry. Once you have eaten, ghrelin levels go down.

Another example is a group of peptide hormones that help regulate blood sugar. While insulin is usually categorized as a protein because it is slightly larger, there are smaller peptide hormones involved in how sugar is taken up by cells. These help make sure your body's tissues get enough energy. If something goes wrong with these signals, it can lead to high or low blood sugar. This is why scientists and doctors care about how these peptide signals work and how to keep them balanced.

Peptide hormones also affect other daily processes, such as waking up and going to sleep. Some peptides interact with the body's internal clock. This clock is located in a part of the brain that senses light and dark, and it uses signals, including peptides, to let other parts of the body know what time it is. This helps keep you in a regular rhythm day after day.

---

3. Immune System Support
Peptides are also involved in the body's defense against germs and harmful substances. Some peptides can directly attack bacteria or viruses. They might poke holes in the outer membrane of bacteria, making it easier for the immune system to remove them. These kinds of peptides are often called antimicrobial peptides, and they are found in many living things, including humans, plants, and insects.

Other peptides help the immune system by sending messages to immune cells. For example, certain peptides might tell immune cells to move to a site of infection or injury. Once there, the immune cells can help remove damaged tissue and fight any harmful invaders. If the immune system needs to calm down after an infection, other peptides can signal this, reducing inflammation so the tissue can heal.

Because of their roles in defense, some researchers want to use peptides as treatments for infections. They hope to find or create peptides that can target germs without harming healthy cells. While there is still much work to be done, peptides hold potential as new tools in the fight against illnesses.

---

4. Tissue Repair and Wound Healing
The body is always carrying out maintenance work. When a tissue is damaged,

such as a cut on your skin, certain peptides may help with healing. They can do this by attracting cells that make new skin or scar tissue to the area. They might also help new blood vessels form so that the healing tissue gets a good supply of nutrients and oxygen.

Some peptides help by reducing swelling around the wound. Others tell cells when it is time to grow or divide so that the damaged tissue can be replaced. Without these signals, healing might be slower or less organized. Because of this, scientists have been studying how to use peptides to help people recover from injuries or surgeries.

For example, there are peptide-based gels that can be applied to wounds. These gels may support the body's own healing processes by creating a protective environment. Some peptides in these gels might push cells to close the wound faster or produce more of the substances that give skin its strength. In this way, the body's natural healing powers get a helping hand.

---

5. Brain and Nerve Function

Peptides also play important roles in the nervous system. Some peptides act as neurotransmitters or neuromodulators. This means they either pass signals from one nerve cell to another or help shape the effects of other signals. For example, certain small peptides might change how we feel pain or pleasure. Others might affect our mood or energy levels.

One peptide that has gained attention is substance P. This peptide is linked to the sensation of pain. When you hurt yourself, substance P is released and helps the signal travel to your brain so you know you are injured. Researchers look at ways to manage substance P to help with certain types of chronic pain. If they can manage how it acts, they might be able to reduce pain in a controlled way.

Certain disorders of the nervous system may involve problems with peptides. That is why some treatments under study focus on stabilizing or changing the levels of particular peptides in the brain. If science can understand these links better, it may help in creating treatments for mood problems or degenerative conditions.

6. Muscle Maintenance and Coordination

Muscles use proteins and peptides to stay strong and flexible. For instance, some peptides help your body move nutrients into muscle cells so they can repair and grow. When you work out, your muscle fibers get small tears, and the body fixes these tears, often building the muscle back stronger than before. Peptides can assist in the repair process by signaling cells to make new proteins or supply energy where it is needed.

In addition, the nerves that tell muscles to contract also rely on peptide messengers. If the communication breaks down, muscles might become weak or unresponsive. By studying these peptides, scientists may find ways to help people who have muscle diseases.

Sometimes, athletes look into peptide supplements to aid recovery. However, this area can be complex because the body's balance of peptides is delicate. Using any kind of supplement without proper care can lead to risks. Peptide research aims to understand how muscle control works at a deep level, so we can keep our muscles working properly.

---

7. Heart and Blood Vessels

Peptides also influence the heart and blood vessels. There are peptide signals that can make blood vessels widen or narrow, helping to regulate blood pressure. If blood pressure is too high, certain peptides might help relax the vessel walls. On the other hand, if blood pressure is too low, other signals might cause the vessels to tighten, bringing the pressure up.

The heart itself can release certain peptides when it is under strain. These peptides might tell the kidneys to get rid of more salt and water, lowering the amount of fluid in the body. As a result, the heart has less work to do. Doctors sometimes measure the levels of these heart-related peptides to see if someone is dealing with heart failure or another heart condition.

Because these peptides are natural regulators of blood pressure and fluid balance, scientists have created medications based on them. By copying or modifying the structure of these peptides, the medicines can help people keep blood pressure at a healthier level. This is just another way that understanding peptides has led to real-world health solutions.

8. Digestive Processes

Peptides in the gut affect how we break down food and absorb nutrients. Some help manage the movement of the digestive tract. Others trigger the release of acids or enzymes that break down food. When you eat, peptide signals tell the stomach to produce acid. They also might tell the pancreas to release enzymes that digest carbohydrates, fats, and proteins.

Additionally, some gut peptides play a part in telling you when you have eaten enough. They send signals to the brain to say, "We are full now." This is connected to hormones like ghrelin mentioned earlier, but there are many other peptides in the gut that have related roles. If these signals are not working properly, a person might feel very hungry or might not feel hungry at all. This can lead to weight issues or nutritional problems.

Gut peptides also interact with the bacteria in your intestine. These bacteria can create or break down certain peptides themselves. In turn, these peptides might influence how the gut barrier works, how the immune cells in the gut behave, and how nutrients are absorbed. Thus, peptides help keep the digestive system in balance.

9. Blood Clotting and Healing

When there is a cut or tear in a blood vessel, the body must quickly patch it up to avoid major blood loss. Peptides can help in this process by aiding in the clotting system. Clotting is complex and involves many proteins, but peptides are there to guide some of these steps. Certain peptides might tell platelets, which are small cells in the blood, to come together and form a plug. Other peptides might help control when clotting should stop, so the clot does not grow too big.

If the clotting process goes wrong, it could lead to a high risk of bleeding or unwanted clots that block blood flow. Researchers look at peptides that control clotting to discover ways to treat conditions where blood does not clot well or clots in the wrong place. For instance, some peptide-based treatments might prevent platelets from sticking together too much, lowering the risk of a dangerous clot. On the flip side, if someone's blood cannot clot, doctors might try to help by giving substances that support clotting signals.

10. Metabolic Balance
Peptides have important jobs in how the body uses energy. Hormones are one example. Some are made of peptides that tell cells how to use or store sugar and fat. If these peptide signals get out of sync, it can lead to issues such as obesity or metabolic disorders.

Scientists are also studying how certain peptides might help people with unstable blood sugar. By improving the signals that lead cells to take in sugar at the right times, the body can maintain a healthier balance of energy. Some peptide-based treatments are approved for managing blood sugar in people with serious problems in this area.

---

11. Skin and Connective Tissue
Skin is not just a covering; it is a living organ that protects us and helps control body temperature. Peptides can help keep skin strong by supporting collagen, elastin, and other structural proteins in the skin. When the skin is damaged by the sun or small injuries, certain peptides may be released to start the repair process. These peptides might tell skin cells to replace damaged parts or produce more of the proteins that help skin stay firm.

Connective tissues are found throughout the body, holding organs and structures in place. They include tendons, ligaments, and layers around organs. Peptides in these tissues can help them remain resilient. If connective tissues break down too easily, it can lead to sprains, tears, or other injuries. By looking at these peptides more closely, scientists hope to understand the best ways to protect or repair connective tissue. Some sports doctors already explore how peptide therapy might help with sports injuries.

---

12. Unique Functions in Different Organs
While we have covered many major roles, it is important to note that peptides can have unique tasks in each organ. For example, in the liver, some peptides assist in processing toxins so they can be removed from the body. In the lungs, certain peptides may help keep airways clear or support healthy tissue. In the kidneys, peptides help control the balance of water and salts. This is linked to how the body keeps blood pressure and fluid levels steady.

In glands, peptides can help release other hormones or substances. In bones, certain peptides are involved in the regular breakdown and rebuilding cycle that keeps bones strong. Each organ may use a variety of peptides, each with a specialized shape and sequence. As you can see, peptides act like small messengers or helpers in nearly every part of the body.

13. How the Body Makes and Regulates Peptides

The body makes peptides using instructions encoded in DNA. First, a larger molecule is made, which can then be cut into smaller peptide pieces. In other cases, the body links amino acids together to form shorter chains right away. Once a peptide is made, it might get changed by enzymes that add or remove certain groups. These changes can make the peptide active or inactive. This is how the body controls when a peptide should do its job.

When a peptide is no longer needed, enzymes break it down into smaller fragments or single amino acids. These parts can be reused to make new proteins or peptides. This cycle allows the body to adapt. If a certain peptide is needed, more can be made. If it is not needed, production can slow down or stop.

14. Balancing Effects and Potential Problems

Even though peptides do good things, they can cause problems if levels get too high or too low. For example, if a peptide that signals swelling is constantly active, the person may end up with chronic inflammation, which can harm organs. If a peptide that tells the body to bring blood sugar down is not working well, that can lead to high blood sugar levels. Balance is key.

The body uses feedback loops to keep peptides in the right range. Feedback loops work like a thermostat. If a peptide signal is too strong, the body might produce a peptide that tells it to slow down. If it is too weak, the body might produce more. This balancing act takes place all the time. Problems arise when feedback loops are broken, which can happen due to genetic issues, infections, or lifestyle factors.

15. Everyday Impact of Peptides

We often do not think about peptides, but they are working constantly behind the scenes. They help us feel hungry or full, keep our skin and muscles in good shape, and guard against germs. They are one reason why the body can quickly respond to challenges. For instance, if you touch a hot surface, signals travel from your hand to your brain and back in a split second, telling you to pull away. Peptides can be part of these rapid communication pathways.

Because peptides are central to so many processes, scientists and doctors keep looking for ways to use them or adjust their levels. Some see them as a way to manage aging, keep muscles in better shape, or help the body heal injuries. Others focus on how peptides might control cravings or how they can be used to make certain therapies safer or more effective.

---

16. Cutting-Edge Research

The study of peptides in the body is a growing field. New peptides are discovered in different tissues, and new roles are found for peptides we already know about. With improved technology, scientists can detect even tiny amounts of peptides in blood or tissue samples. They can also create synthetic peptides in the lab to learn how changing one amino acid affects what a peptide can do. This helps them understand how to design peptide-based medicines that target specific issues.

For instance, researchers might adjust the structure of a known peptide so it lasts longer in the bloodstream. That way, a person would not need as many doses of a medicine based on that peptide. In other cases, they might add a small chemical group that helps the peptide stick to a certain tissue, like the liver or the heart. With each new experiment, we learn more about how to direct peptide actions in precise ways.

---

17. Practical Examples

1. **Skin Creams and Serums**: Some beauty products have peptides that claim to support collagen in the skin. While the effect can depend on how deeply these peptides can get into the skin, some people find them helpful for firmness or tone.

2. **Sports Formulas**: Certain products for sports performance include peptides that are said to help with muscle repair. Though some athletes may explore these, it is important to remember that science is still looking into the long-term safety of many peptide supplements.
3. **Medical Uses**: Peptide-based medicines exist for conditions like diabetes or hormone imbalances. These medicines can help people control blood sugar or replace low hormone levels. They must be prescribed by a doctor and come with instructions on how to use them correctly.
4. **Research Tools**: Scientists use peptides to map out how proteins in cells interact. By designing a peptide that mimics part of a protein, they can see how other molecules bind or respond. This can help reveal the details of important interactions that keep cells alive and healthy.

---

18. Why Peptides Are Important

Peptides stand out because they can be made and broken down quite fast, making them good messengers for quick signals. They also tend to have fewer unwanted effects than some other substances, partly because they are recognized and cleared by the body naturally. This does not mean peptides are free from risks. Each case must be studied to ensure that a specific peptide is safe and does what it is supposed to do.

From managing hunger to protecting against microbes, peptides help keep the body working smoothly. Without them, many processes would slow down or stop. This is why scientists from many fields—medicine, biology, nutrition, and others—are fascinated by peptides. They hope to learn how to use them in new ways to help with diseases, improve overall health, or even help solve some age-related issues.

---

19. Big Picture of Peptide Roles

Overall, peptides make things run more smoothly in the body. They act as signals, regulators, and helpers in:

- **Communication**: Linking cells and organs together
- **Defense**: Supporting the immune system
- **Repair**: Helping tissues after injury
- **Energy**: Managing how the body uses nutrients

- **Growth**: Guiding normal development and maintenance
- **Balance**: Keeping hormones and other signals within healthy limits

By carrying out these tasks, peptides prove just how valuable short chains of amino acids can be.

---

20. Looking Ahead

In future research, we may see more and more peptide-based approaches for health issues. Since peptides can be very specific, doctors might be able to give patients personalized peptides that only affect the tissue or cells that need help. This could reduce side effects that come from treatments that affect the entire body. There is also interest in using peptides to manage problems like antibiotic resistance. If we can design peptides that target harmful bacteria in a new way, we might avoid some of the problems seen with older drugs.

In the next chapter, we will compare peptides with proteins to understand their differences more clearly. This will show why peptides can sometimes do things that proteins cannot, and vice versa. By knowing how peptides stand apart, we can see why they are useful and how they fit into the larger picture of biology.

That wraps up our discussion of peptides and their role in the body. These small chains are active in many tasks, from your head down to your toes. Though they might seem simple at first, their ability to help regulate and guide processes in nearly every organ makes them worth understanding.

Chapter 4: Proteins vs. Peptides

Peptides and proteins can both be made from amino acids. In many ways, peptides are like small versions of proteins. However, there are important differences that set them apart, especially in how they are structured, how big they are, and what they do in the body. This chapter will look at those differences in depth.

---

1. Size and Length
The most obvious difference is size. A peptide is typically shorter, often defined as having up to 50 amino acids. A protein is usually longer than that, sometimes with hundreds or even thousands of amino acids. Because proteins are bigger, they can fold into complex shapes with multiple layers of structure. Peptides may have only a simple chain shape or a small loop.

That said, there is no single rule that says, "At exactly 50 amino acids, a chain must be called a protein." Some people might say a chain with 40 amino acids is still a peptide, while another person might call it a small protein. But it is generally accepted that proteins are larger and peptides are smaller.

---

2. Structural Complexity
Proteins often have multiple levels of structure. Scientists describe these as primary, secondary, tertiary, and sometimes quaternary structures:

- **Primary**: The amino acid sequence.
- **Secondary**: Shapes like alpha helices or beta sheets that form along the chain due to hydrogen bonds.
- **Tertiary**: How the entire chain folds into a 3D shape.
- **Quaternary**: How multiple folded chains fit together to make a larger complex.

Peptides may have less complex folding because they are shorter. They might adopt a simple coil or a small loop structure. Some do form secondary structures, but they do not usually have the large-scale folding patterns of bigger proteins. Because peptides often lack the extensive folding of proteins, they can move through certain tissues more easily. They also might be broken down faster, because it can be simpler for enzymes to reach and clip the shorter chain.

---

3. Function in the Body

Proteins have a huge range of jobs, including forming the structural components of muscle and skin (like collagen and other connective tissues), moving molecules around the body (like hemoglobin carrying oxygen), acting as enzymes that speed up chemical reactions, and sending signals as hormones. Peptides, while also important for signaling, are often best known for their role as messengers that pass instructions between cells. They can also help with defense (such as antimicrobial peptides), growth, digestion, and other tasks.

Because proteins can be very large, they can form structures like hair, nails, and the cytoskeleton inside cells. Peptides, being smaller, rarely form big structural frameworks. Instead, they specialize in rapid signaling or specific, targeted actions. That said, there are a few mid-size peptides that serve as building blocks in bigger complexes.

---

4. Formation and Synthesis

Both peptides and proteins come from amino acids joined by peptide bonds. In living organisms, these are typically made following instructions in the DNA. The process involves a few main steps:

1. **Transcription**: DNA is copied into messenger RNA (mRNA).
2. **Translation**: The cell reads the mRNA and assembles amino acids in the correct order to form a chain.
3. **Folding or Modifications**: The chain might fold, or enzymes might make changes such as adding carbohydrate groups or cutting out sections.

For proteins, these steps can be more involved. The chain can be hundreds of amino acids long, and the folding can be very complex. Peptides are shorter and may not need as many steps to become functional. Sometimes, a large protein is made and then cut into smaller pieces that function as peptides. In other cases, the body creates a peptide directly by assembling a short chain from the start.

In labs, scientists can also make peptides. This is simpler for short chains than for large proteins. Synthetic peptide production involves joining protected amino acids one by one. Once the chain is complete, it can be "deprotected," giving a finished peptide. While larger proteins can be made in a lab as well, they usually require cell-based expression systems because the chain is too large or folds in a complex way that demands the help of cellular machinery.

---

5. Stability

Proteins, due to their size and intricate folding, often have regions that protect them from enzymes that break down amino acids. They can also have stable bonds between parts of the chain, such as disulfide bridges. Peptides, being smaller, can be broken down more quickly. This breakdown is not always a bad thing. In the body, it can help regulate how long a signaling peptide remains active.

However, if someone wants a peptide to stay active longer, they might alter its structure. For example, scientists may replace certain amino acids with synthetic ones that the body's enzymes do not recognize as easily. This can make the peptide more stable. Proteins can also be modified for stability, but they may need more support to maintain their correct shape.

---

6. Delivery in the Body

Another contrast is how peptides and proteins can be given as treatments. Many protein-based drugs must be injected because they are too large and fragile to survive the acidic environment of the stomach. Peptides often have the same problem, though sometimes their small size allows for creative delivery methods, such as nasal sprays or skin patches.

Proteins, due to their size, may not pass through cell membranes easily. Peptides can sometimes slip through membranes more effectively, although not all peptides can do this. Some peptides need a special carrier to help them cross. Researchers keep working on new ways to deliver both proteins and peptides so that they can reach their target tissues without being destroyed along the way.

---

7. Examples of Proteins vs. Examples of Peptides

- **Proteins**:
    1. **Hemoglobin**: Carries oxygen in red blood cells. It is made of four large protein chains.
    2. **Collagen**: Found in skin, bones, and connective tissues. Gives these tissues strength.
    3. **Enzymes** (like amylase or lactase): Speed up chemical reactions that help break down food or perform other tasks in cells.
    4. **Antibodies**: Large proteins that help the immune system recognize and remove harmful invaders.
- **Peptides**:
    1. **Bradykinin**: Helps manage blood vessel widening.
    2. **Angiotensin II**: Influences blood pressure and fluid balance.
    3. **Oxytocin**: Known for roles in social bonding and certain bodily functions, such as helping the uterus contract during childbirth.
    4. **Antimicrobial Peptides**: Defend against germs by disrupting their membranes.

These examples show how proteins often have large, heavy tasks, while peptides often serve in rapid signaling or tight control of certain body processes.

---

8. Folding and Function

Because proteins fold in detailed ways, they often create specific "active sites." These sites are like pockets or grooves where reactions take place. For example, an enzyme's active site is shaped just right to grab a certain molecule and transform it. Proteins can also have separate sections called domains, each with its own role. This level of complexity is part of what allows proteins to do so many varied tasks.

Peptides do not usually have multiple domains. They might fold into a small loop or coil, but they rarely have distinct parts that function independently. They are also less likely to have large interior regions. Instead, peptides might have one continuous surface that can attach to a receptor or membrane. Some peptides do fold into stable patterns like alpha helices, but they are generally still simpler than full-sized proteins.

9. Industrial and Commercial Uses

In industries, proteins are used in tasks like washing clothes (enzymes to break down stains), making foods (enzymes to help process cheese or bread), and many other processes. Peptides can also be used commercially, though typically in more specialized areas. For instance, certain peptide-based products might be developed for skin care. They might help with firming skin or reducing swelling. Other peptide products might aim to protect crops from pests, acting as safe and natural insect controls.

Proteins sometimes serve as bulk materials. Gelatin is a form of partially broken-down collagen. It can form gels used in foods or capsules for supplements. Peptides can be found in protein hydrolysates, which are mixtures of smaller chains used to enrich foods or feed products. These products have peptides that might be easier to digest than whole proteins.

10. Research Approaches

When studying proteins in the lab, scientists often use methods like X-ray crystallography or cryo-electron microscopy to see the shape. These are advanced techniques that can provide detailed images of how atoms are arranged. With peptides, some of these methods still apply, but it can be faster or simpler to analyze the structure, given the smaller size.

Scientists who want to test how a peptide works may synthesize it in different forms, each with small changes in the amino acid sequence. They can see which version binds better to a receptor or lasts longer in the bloodstream. This process can lead to a new peptide-based therapy. Meanwhile, large protein research may need entire cell factories where bacteria or yeast produce the protein, followed by complex purification steps.

11. Legal and Regulatory Matters

When peptides are used in medicine, they go through a regulation process similar to what proteins go through. However, they are often quicker to develop because of their simpler structure. Still, the safety and effectiveness of a peptide-based product must be carefully tested. Regulatory agencies must check that a new peptide drug does not cause harmful side effects and that it does what the maker says it does.

Proteins, especially those made by genetic engineering, also face strict checks. Because proteins can be large and sometimes lead to allergic reactions, they require detailed testing. Some protein-based drugs, called biologics, can take many years of research before they are allowed for public use. Peptide drugs may sometimes move through trials more quickly if they are easier to produce and verify.

---

12. Breakdown in the Body

Once a protein or peptide has done its job, it is usually broken down by enzymes into amino acids, which can then be reused. The smaller size of peptides means they are often broken down faster, unless they have special features like loops or modified amino acids. Proteins might take longer to break down, partly because they have places that enzymes cannot easily reach.

Because peptides tend to have a shorter life in the bloodstream, some see this as a downside for therapy. Patients might have to take more frequent doses. On the plus side, if a peptide causes unwanted effects, these might not last very long once the peptide is removed or broken down. Proteins, being larger and possibly more stable, can remain in the body longer, which might be good for long-term treatment but could be bad if side effects appear.

---

13. Cost and Accessibility

Developing new proteins, especially large ones, can be expensive. It might involve engineering cells to produce the protein in large quantities, then purifying it. Peptides can be cheaper to produce synthetically in some cases, especially if they are not too long. However, the cost can go up if complicated modifications are required to keep them stable or help them reach the right part of the body.

This difference in production costs can affect the price of treatments. Some protein-based treatments, such as certain cancer drugs or rare disease therapies, can be very expensive. Some peptide-based drugs might be less costly, though not always. It depends on how the drug is made and how complex it is to store and transport.

14. Use in Diagnostics
Proteins and peptides can both be used in diagnostic tests. For instance, doctors might measure the level of a certain protein in the blood to see if you have an infection. They might also measure specific peptides to find out if you are at risk for heart failure or if your endocrine system is working properly.

Proteins can serve as markers for diseases, like how prostate-specific antigen (PSA) can be a marker for prostate problems. Peptides can also be markers, such as certain peptide fragments that appear in the blood when a tissue is breaking down. Knowing the levels of these proteins or peptides can help doctors diagnose conditions sooner and treat them more effectively.

---

15. Food and Digestion
Proteins in our diets, such as those from meat, beans, or dairy, are often broken down into smaller chains of amino acids (peptides) and then into single amino acids. The body then rebuilds these amino acids into the specific proteins or peptides it needs. Some small peptides in food may be absorbed directly if they are stable enough.

Fermented foods might have higher levels of small peptides because the bacteria or yeasts produce enzymes that break down proteins. Some of these peptides may have health benefits, like supporting digestion or having mild effects on blood pressure. Research into how dietary peptides help the body is still ongoing, but it is an interesting area that sits at the intersection of nutrition and biology.

---

16. Interchange Between Peptides and Proteins
Sometimes, the body makes a large protein and then cuts it into smaller peptides that do various tasks. In other cases, the body might need to link peptides together or extend them to form bigger proteins. This means that peptides and proteins are part of the same overall system: both are made of amino acids, and the body can reshape these amino acids into different forms as needed.

For example, a large precursor protein might stay inactive until a part of it is removed, revealing an active peptide. This is a way the body can store a hormone in an inactive form and then switch it on only when needed. The same principle can work in reverse: the body might bind smaller chains together to form a bigger structure. In both directions, the process is guided by enzymes that know exactly where to cut or join the chain.

---

17. Medical Treatments and Research Directions

Proteins often make up treatments like enzyme replacements, monoclonal antibodies, or hormones like insulin. Peptides are gaining ground as medicines too. Scientists see a bright future for peptide drugs that can target specific receptors. One benefit is that peptides can often be tailored to work only where needed, lowering the chance of widespread effects.

At the same time, researchers are exploring new ways to make proteins more stable or get them into cells that were once thought unreachable. Nanotechnology, for example, might help "package" proteins so they can move through the bloodstream safely. Similar methods might also help peptides survive longer. As these technologies evolve, the boundary between what is possible with proteins and peptides may change, allowing for new therapies we have not imagined yet.

---

18. Suitability for Different Tasks

When deciding whether to use a protein or a peptide for a certain role, scientists consider factors like:

- **Size Needed**: Do we need a large structure with multiple functions, or a small messenger?
- **Delivery Method**: Will it be swallowed, injected, or applied to the skin?
- **Stability**: Does it need to stay active for a long time, or is a short burst of activity enough?
- **Complexity of Action**: Does the molecule need several active sites or just one?

Proteins might be chosen if they need to carry out a complex reaction or form part of a physical structure. Peptides might be better if a quick, targeted signal is all that is required, or if the therapy requires a molecule that can move quickly through tissues.

19. Everyday Examples

In everyday life, you might not think much about whether something is a protein or a peptide, but both are present. The proteins in your meal are broken down into peptides during digestion. If you use a skin product that has "collagen peptides" on the label, that is a reference to smaller chains derived from collagen. If you hear about research on a new "peptide drug," that is a clue it is likely to be smaller than a standard protein-based drug like a full antibody.

When washing clothes, enzymes in detergents are proteins. If you have leftover food that grows mold, some peptides could be in that mold, acting to break down the food. Nature uses these molecules everywhere, and the difference usually comes down to how many amino acids they have and how they fold.

---

20. Summary of Key Points

- **Length**: Proteins are bigger, peptides are smaller.
- **Folding**: Proteins often have complex shapes, peptides are usually simpler.
- **Function**: Proteins can be structural or enzymatic, peptides often serve as signals or smaller helpers.
- **Stability**: Proteins can be more stable; peptides tend to be broken down faster.
- **Synthesis**: Both come from amino acids joined by peptide bonds, but proteins require more extensive steps for proper folding.
- **Uses**: Both are vital in medicine, industry, and biology.

Understanding these differences shows why a problem might call for a peptide-based solution rather than a protein-based one, or the other way around. Some situations need a big, stable molecule with multiple functions, while others need a small, precise messenger that can be created and removed quickly.

With this clear distinction in mind, we can better appreciate how peptides and proteins each have unique strengths. In the next chapters, we will see how peptides are used in health-related areas, skin care, and beyond. This knowledge of their differences will help us see why certain applications lean more toward peptides while others rely on full-sized proteins.

Through all of this, it is important to remember that peptides and proteins do not exist in isolation. They both emerge from amino acids in living systems, and the body often switches between them as needed. This combination of flexibility and specialization is part of what makes life so adaptable and diverse. By paying attention to these details, scientists and doctors can tailor peptides or proteins to solve a wide range of problems and improve overall well-being.

Chapter 5: Therapeutic Uses of Peptides

Peptides have become an important part of modern medicine. Scientists and doctors often use them in treatments for diseases and health conditions. Because peptides can be designed for specific targets, they can help with problems that were difficult to manage in the past. In this chapter, we will look at several areas where peptides are used or studied for use in therapy. We will also look at the reasons why peptides can be so helpful, and some of the challenges involved in making and using them.

1. Overview of Peptide Therapies

Peptides are small chains of amino acids. Because of their size, they often have fewer side effects than bigger molecules, like large proteins or complicated chemical drugs. They can be cleared from the body more quickly once they have done their job. Sometimes, they do need help staying stable in the bloodstream, but researchers have found ways to protect them by making slight changes to their structure or combining them with other substances.

A key benefit is that peptides can be very specific. They attach to certain cell receptors or fit into certain spots inside the body, much like a key that only works for one lock. This makes them less likely to accidentally attach to the wrong target. By being so specific, a peptide may lead to fewer problems throughout the rest of the body. Of course, every drug or therapy can have side effects, but with peptides, it may be easier to limit them by focusing on particular tissues.

Some peptide treatments have been approved for regular use, while others are still being tested. In recent years, many research labs have begun to explore new ways to create, modify, and deliver peptides, leading to a wide range of possible therapies.

2. Hormone and Metabolic Disorders

One of the earliest peptide therapies involved hormones. In fact, insulin, which is often labeled as a protein, is sometimes discussed alongside peptides because it is made up of amino-acid chains. Insulin helps regulate blood sugar and is a key treatment for people who have trouble producing enough insulin on their own.

Beyond insulin, there are other peptide therapies for conditions related to blood sugar. Some peptides help the body release more insulin after meals, or slow the emptying of the stomach so that blood sugar does not spike too quickly. These therapies can make day-to-day life easier for people who have ongoing problems with sugar control. By focusing on the signals that manage how the body uses sugar, peptides can help keep it within a safer range.

Other metabolic disorders may also benefit from peptide-based treatments. For example, scientists are studying peptides that affect how the body stores or burns fat. The idea is that if you can safely guide the body's signals, you might help people keep a healthier weight or avoid complications related to too much stored fat. While these ideas are still being tested in many cases, they highlight the potential of peptides to fine-tune the body's own signals instead of simply shutting them on or off.

---

3. Autoimmune Conditions

In autoimmune conditions, the immune system mistakenly attacks the body's own cells. One aim of peptide therapy is to create treatments that calm down these harmful immune responses without stopping the immune system from doing its normal protective work. Some peptides can attach to immune cells and guide their activity. Rather than silencing the entire immune system, these peptides might block only the signals linked to harmful attacks.

For instance, in certain conditions where cells in joints or tissues are attacked, a peptide might be designed to block the interaction that triggers that attack. Because peptides are so specific, they can sometimes block the harmful activity while leaving useful immune functions alone. This is different from broader treatments that make the entire immune system weaker, which can leave people open to infections.

This area of research involves careful checking. If a peptide does not attach strongly enough, it will not have the desired effect. If it sticks around too long, it might cause unwanted changes. Still, the idea of using peptides to guide the immune system continues to show promise, and more clinical trials are looking at these therapies.

---

4. Chronic Pain and Neurological Issues

Some peptides may help people who have trouble with pain that lasts for a long time. When the body senses pain, it sends signals through nerves to the brain. Certain small peptides act as messengers in this pathway. If these messengers are too active, a person might feel excessive pain, even when the injury is minor. If scientists can use a peptide that blocks or changes these signals, they may reduce pain.

An example is the research on substance P, a peptide linked to pain signals. By blocking substance P in specific ways, some experimental treatments hope to prevent pain from becoming overwhelming. Other peptides work on different nerve pathways to shift how pain is processed. While many of these ideas are still in testing, the field of pain research is very interested in peptides because they can be targeted to certain nerve channels or receptors.

In neurological conditions, there are also hopes that peptides might protect nerve cells from damage or help them repair. Some peptides encourage growth in nerve tissue, while others might stop harmful processes that break down nerve cells. If scientists can get these peptides where they need to go—often across the blood-brain barrier—it may open up new treatment paths for conditions that have been difficult to manage.

---

5. Fighting Infections

Many organisms, including humans, make antimicrobial peptides to protect against germs. These peptides can kill or disable bacteria, viruses, or fungi by disrupting their outer layers or blocking certain steps in their life cycle. Some of these natural antimicrobial peptides are being developed into medicines, either by copying them exactly or by changing them slightly for extra stability.

The need for new ways to fight infections is huge. Over time, some germs have become resistant to older antibiotics. Peptide-based treatments might attack germs differently, making it harder for them to develop resistance. However, these treatments still have hurdles, such as how to make the peptides last long enough to do their work or how to deliver them to infected tissues without being broken down too soon.

Research groups around the world are testing many antimicrobial peptides in lab dishes and animal models. Some show strong results in targeting infections that do not respond well to standard antibiotics. With more testing, these peptides might reach human trials and become new tools for doctors.

---

6. Cancer Treatments

Cancer is a complex condition where cells multiply out of control. Standard treatments like chemotherapy can harm healthy cells along with the cancer cells. Peptides offer a targeted approach: they can be designed to attach to markers found mostly on tumor cells. Once they lock onto these markers, they might block signals that let the cancer grow, or they might guide drugs directly to the tumor.

For example, a peptide might be linked to a toxin or a radioactive particle. If the peptide only binds to tumor cells, it can bring the destructive agent right where it is needed, sparing healthy cells around it. This is called peptide-drug conjugation. Another approach uses peptides to prompt the immune system to target the cancer more strongly. By directing the body's own defenses, the treatment might shrink tumors or slow their growth.

Still, creating cancer-targeting peptides can be difficult. Tumors vary in their markers, and they can change over time. Also, the peptides must be tested carefully to ensure they do not gather in healthy tissues. Trials are ongoing, and some peptide-based cancer drugs have moved into later stages of clinical testing. The hope is that such therapies will lead to more precise ways to treat different cancer types.

7. Tissue Repair and Regeneration

When someone has a serious wound or tissue damage, the body's own healing processes might need extra help. Certain peptides encourage cells to regrow or form new blood vessels. By placing these peptides in the injured area, for example in a gel or bandage, doctors might help the tissue recover faster. In burns or large wounds, healing can be slow and prone to infection. Peptide-based treatments aim to make the environment more favorable for tissue repair.

For cartilage or bone problems, some experimental therapies use peptides to lure special cells to the damage site. These cells can then build new tissue. Cartilage does not heal easily on its own, so any approach that can assist this process is useful. The same goes for injuries to muscles or tendons. Animal studies have shown that certain peptides can speed up healing, but more human trials are needed to confirm safety and long-term effects.

---

8. Heart and Blood Vessel Support

Some peptide-based therapies help with heart conditions. The heart releases certain peptides when it is under strain, and doctors can measure them to see how stressed the heart is. In terms of treatment, there are peptides that cause blood vessels to widen, lowering blood pressure. Others may guide the kidneys to manage fluid levels in the body, helping ease the strain on the heart.

Scientists have also looked into peptides that prevent unwanted blood clots. These peptides might interfere with the steps that lead platelets to stick together. If used carefully, they could reduce the risk of stroke or heart attack. However, the same therapy could raise bleeding risks, so dosing and timing become very important.

Peptides might also help the heart tissue recover after an injury, such as a heart attack. By encouraging new blood vessels to grow or telling damaged cells to repair themselves, peptides could lower the damage. This area of study is still ongoing, but it shows how small molecules can have a strong effect on organ repair.

9. Delivery Challenges

While peptides have many uses, delivering them properly can be tricky. The body has enzymes that break down proteins and peptides. If a peptide is taken by mouth, it might be destroyed in the stomach before it can help. That is why many peptide-based drugs need to be injected or delivered in another special way, such as a nasal spray or a skin patch.

Researchers tackle this issue by making small changes to the peptide structure so that enzymes do not recognize it as easily. They might replace an amino acid with a lab-made version, or they might attach the peptide to a larger molecule like polyethylene glycol (PEG). These changes can keep the peptide active for a longer time and allow it to reach the tissues that need it.

Another challenge is making sure the peptide goes where it is intended. If a peptide aims to fix a problem in the brain, it must cross the blood-brain barrier, which is difficult for many substances. Scientists try to solve this by adding features to the peptide that let it pass through cells lining the blood vessels in the brain. Even then, it can be an uphill task to get enough of the peptide to the right spot.

---

10. Safety and Side Effects

Although peptides are often seen as safer than some other treatments, they are not entirely without risks. A peptide might target a receptor in one area of the body, but the same receptor might exist in another area. If it binds there, unexpected effects could happen. This is why careful testing is required to confirm that a peptide therapy will do more good than harm.

Patients can also develop allergic reactions to peptide drugs. This is less common than with certain bigger proteins, but it can happen. Dosing is another concern. Because peptides can break down or be cleared quickly, patients might need more frequent doses or a long-acting version. Too much of a certain peptide could lead to harmful changes in blood pressure, immune function, or other processes.

Regulators require that new peptide therapies go through stages of testing, starting in lab dishes, then in animals, and finally in humans. Each step checks for potential dangers. If the peptide makes it through these steps successfully, it can be approved for use. Even after approval, doctors and researchers keep track of how patients respond to see if any rare issues show up over time.

---

11. Examples of Approved Peptide Therapies

Many peptides have already been approved in different parts of the world. While the exact list changes as new ones are added and others are retired, here are some examples of peptide-based treatments you might come across:

1. **Glucagon-Like Peptide-1 (GLP-1) Receptor Agonists**: These help with sugar control in people who have trouble managing blood glucose levels on their own. They slow down digestion and boost insulin release.
2. **Liraglutide**: A modified version of a natural peptide that helps manage weight and blood sugar in certain individuals. It is designed to last longer in the bloodstream than the natural version.
3. **Buserelin or Leuprolide**: These are peptide-based drugs that affect hormone release and can be used for hormone-sensitive conditions. They work by first boosting, then reducing hormone signals in a controlled way.
4. **Calcitonin**: This peptide helps manage calcium levels in the body and can be used to treat osteoporosis. It slows down the cells that break down bone tissue.
5. **Desmopressin**: A peptide that helps the body manage water balance. It can be used for conditions where someone loses too much fluid or cannot hold on to fluids well.

These are just a few examples out of many. Each one went through years of research and testing to show it is both safe and effective for a certain group of patients.

---

12. Personalized Medicine Possibilities

Because peptides can be designed and changed, they fit well with the idea of personalized medicine. This is the approach where treatments are matched to an individual's genetic makeup and specific health needs. If doctors find that a patient's cells have a certain receptor or a unique set of markers, they might be able to design a peptide that targets just those cells.

While this idea is still mostly in the research stage, it shows how flexible peptide therapies can be. One day, a patient with a certain type of cancer might receive a tailor-made peptide that attaches to markers found only on that tumor. Someone with a genetic condition might get a peptide that fixes a signal that is not working properly. Although this is still a hope for the future, studies in labs are moving in that direction.

13. Cost and Accessibility

Making peptides can be cheaper than making large protein drugs, but it is still not always simple. Synthetic processes require special equipment and chemicals, and if the peptide needs special modifications, the cost can go up. Additionally, the research and clinical trials behind each new therapy can cost a lot, which can lead to high prices once a peptide therapy is approved.

Over time, as technology improves and more companies produce peptide treatments, costs may go down. However, it remains important for health systems to find ways to make these therapies accessible. Many serious conditions could be improved or managed with peptide treatments, but if the cost is too high, not everyone will benefit.

14. The Future of Peptide-Based Therapies

Researchers continue to find new ways to use peptides in medicine. Some labs use computers to design peptides from scratch, aiming to fit certain receptors perfectly. Others search nature for novel peptides in plants, marine life, or microscopic organisms. These natural peptides might already have the ability to fight bacteria or reduce swelling, and scientists can study them to see if they could become new drugs.

Improvements in drug delivery methods, such as nanocarriers or smart patches, might also push peptides into new areas of therapy. If it becomes easier to protect peptides from the gut or to guide them past barriers like the blood-brain barrier, we might see a surge in peptide treatments for problems that are currently hard to fix. With each year, more groups publish studies showing interesting peptide findings, so it seems likely that these small chains of amino acids will keep playing a bigger role in health care.

---

15. Collaboration Across Fields

Developing a peptide drug often needs experts from many areas. Chemists figure out how to make or modify the peptide. Biologists check how it behaves in cells and in animals. Medical doctors run clinical trials to see if it is safe and helpful. Regulatory experts ensure the therapy meets safety rules. Manufacturing teams figure out how to make enough of the peptide at a good price. Finally, pharmacists and nurses help patients use the new therapy correctly.

Because of this teamwork, peptide drugs are part of a broader web of innovation. Government agencies, universities, hospitals, and private companies all work together to take a peptide from the lab bench to the clinic. This process might take many years, but each success can change the lives of people with serious health problems.

---

16. Key Takeaways

1. **Specificity**: Peptides can be designed to attach to certain receptors, reducing side effects.
2. **Wide Applications**: They are studied for many health issues, including metabolic disorders, immune problems, infections, and cancer.
3. **Delivery Issues**: The body's enzymes can break down peptides, so new delivery systems or structural changes are needed.
4. **Regulatory Oversight**: Peptide therapies undergo a strict approval process to ensure they are safe and effective.
5. **Future Potential**: Ongoing research in peptide design, delivery, and discovery hints at more treatments on the way.

Therapeutic uses of peptides are likely to keep expanding. Even though there are hurdles related to cost, stability, and targeted delivery, these can often be addressed through careful science. As new discoveries are made, it is possible that more people with hard-to-treat conditions will gain access to helpful peptide-based treatments.

That concludes our look at how peptides are used to help the body. Next, we will shift our focus from medical therapy to how peptides are applied in everyday beauty routines, with a special look at skin care.

Chapter 6: Peptides in Skin Care

Peptides have become popular in the world of skin care. Many product labels highlight them to catch the attention of consumers who hope for healthier, smoother-looking skin. In this chapter, we will look at what peptides can do for the skin, why they are included in creams and serums, and what science says about their effectiveness. We will also discuss other factors involved in skin health, so we can see that peptides are only one piece of a bigger picture.

---

1. Understanding the Skin's Structure

The skin has multiple layers. The outermost layer is the epidermis, which acts as a shield against germs and helps keep moisture inside. Beneath that is the dermis, where we find collagen, elastin, and other important fibers. Collagen provides firmness, while elastin allows the skin to stretch and return to its normal shape. Deeper still is the subcutaneous layer, which has fat and connective tissues.

Age, sun exposure, and other factors can change the structure of the skin, leading to dryness, lines, and other visible signs. The reason many beauty products focus on collagen is that lower levels of collagen and elastin can affect how skin looks and feels. Because peptides are tied to the production and arrangement of these proteins, some people hope that applying the right peptides can help the skin in various ways.

---

2. Why Peptides in Skin Care?

Peptides can act like small messengers, telling cells to do certain tasks. For instance, there are signal peptides that give a message to skin cells to produce more collagen or other structural proteins. If these peptides manage to get through the skin's surface and bind to the right cells, they might help support the normal processes that keep skin strong.

Some skin care brands also include carrier peptides that help deliver key minerals or other substances to skin cells. The idea is that the peptide can bind to a mineral, such as copper, and then transport it where it is needed. Copper can be important for collagen production, so these products claim to encourage healthy-looking skin by providing both the mineral and the messenger.

Additionally, certain peptides might calm the look of wrinkles by signaling to muscles or by interfering with the steps that cause deep lines. While this does not cause the same effect as medical procedures, the right peptide might help soften the appearance of lines over time. Of course, each peptide is unique, and not all peptides work the same way. The variety of peptides in beauty products shows how many different strategies brands are trying.

3. Types of Peptides in Skin Care

Skin care lines may talk about different families of peptides. Even though the names can be long and complicated, it can help to know the general categories:

1. **Signal Peptides**: These are meant to communicate with skin cells to produce more collagen, elastin, or other substances that support the skin. They often have names that reference the type of protein they affect.
2. **Carrier Peptides**: They bind and carry trace elements like copper or magnesium. The skin uses these elements in producing enzymes or building blocks for collagen.
3. **Enzyme-Inhibitor Peptides**: They might reduce the breakdown of collagen by blocking enzymes that degrade skin fibers. If collagen is not broken down as quickly, it can help maintain firmer-looking skin.
4. **Neurotransmitter-Inhibitor Peptides**: Some peptides claim to reduce the signals that tighten facial muscles, aiming to lessen lines. They are sometimes called "topical relaxers," though their effect is usually mild compared to clinical injections.

Each category serves a different purpose. Some brands combine multiple peptides in a single product, hoping to address various skin concerns at once.

4. Do Peptides Really Help Skin?

Research suggests that certain peptides can make a difference when applied on the skin, but results can vary based on multiple factors:

- **Concentration**: The product must contain a sufficient amount of the peptide. If it is too low, the effect may be minimal.

- **Delivery Method**: Peptides must reach the cells in the deeper layers. If the product only stays on the surface, it might not have a strong effect.
- **Stability**: Some peptides are fragile and can break down easily in the jar or on the skin. They might also lose effectiveness if exposed to air or light.
- **Combination with Other Ingredients**: Sometimes peptides work best when paired with substances like antioxidants, hyaluronic acid, or vitamins that support skin health.

In some studies, topical application of certain peptides led to improvements in skin firmness or the appearance of fine lines. However, these studies often use specific formulas under controlled conditions. Real-world results can be influenced by a person's overall routine, diet, sun exposure, age, and genetics. Even so, many consumers report noticing softer or smoother-looking skin when they use peptide products regularly.

5. Limitations and Common Myths

Peptides in skin care are not magical. Some advertisements might make big claims, suggesting that a certain peptide can transform the skin almost overnight. Realistically, even the best products need time to show results, and they cannot fully replace medical treatments. In fact, if a product promises to instantly remove wrinkles, it might be using ingredients that simply tighten the top layer of the skin temporarily rather than increasing collagen.

Another point to remember is that peptides alone cannot fix damage from heavy sun exposure, smoking, or an unhealthy lifestyle. Skin health depends on protecting it from UV rays, drinking enough water, and getting nutrients that help the skin repair itself. Peptides can be a helpful part of a broader routine, but they are not the only factor. Also, not every product that claims to have peptides will contain the type or amount that can make a real difference.

6. Product Forms and Labels

Peptide-based products often come in creams, serums, or lotions. Serums are usually more concentrated, which might give the peptides a better chance to work. Moisturizers that include peptides also provide hydration, which is important for keeping skin plump. When looking at labels, you might see ingredient names like "palmitoyl pentapeptide," "acetyl hexapeptide," or "copper tripeptide." These names refer to the specific sequence of amino acids and possible added chemical groups.

It is useful to remember that not all peptide products are alike. Concentration matters, as does the product's design. A properly formulated serum will try to keep the peptide stable and ensure that it is delivered past the surface. Some products might have packaging that protects the ingredients from air and light. Others might have clear containers that allow light to pass through, which could weaken certain peptides over time.

7. Examples of Common Skin Care Peptides

1. **Palmitoyl Pentapeptide-4**: Often marketed to support collagen, this peptide has been studied for its ability to reduce the look of fine lines.
2. **Copper Tripeptide-1**: This peptide has copper attached, which can help with collagen production. It is sometimes included in products that aim to promote a smoother, more even appearance.
3. **Acetyl Hexapeptide-8**: Sometimes described as a surface-level muscle signal blocker. It aims to soften the look of expression lines by dampening certain signals.
4. **Palmitoyl Tripeptide-1**: May help with the visible signs of aging by boosting collagen and other structural elements in the skin.

These are just a few examples among many. Each peptide has a specific structure that aims to address a particular aspect of skin health.

8. How to Use Peptide Products

If you decide to include a peptide-based product in your routine, consider these tips:

- **Cleansing**: Wash your face with a gentle cleanser before applying peptides. This removes oil and dirt so the peptides can reach your skin more easily.

- **Order of Application**: Thinner, water-based serums or lotions should go on before heavier creams or oils. If you use a toner or essence, that usually comes before the serum.
- **Sun Protection**: Many peptides can help with overall skin appearance, but they cannot protect you from the sun's harmful rays. Use sunscreen daily to keep skin damage from building up.
- **Be Patient**: It often takes weeks to notice changes. Keep an eye on how your skin responds, and do not switch products too frequently.
- **Check for Irritation**: Some people may be sensitive to certain peptides or other ingredients in a formula. If you notice redness or discomfort, stop using the product or try a gentler version.

---

9. Combining Peptides with Other Ingredients

Peptides can work well alongside other substances that help the skin. For example, combining peptides with antioxidants like vitamin C can help reduce the effects of free radicals. Vitamin C also helps in collagen building, so it complements the action of certain signal peptides.

Another common partner is hyaluronic acid, which can help hydrate the skin. When the skin is well-hydrated, it is more receptive to active ingredients and also appears smoother. Niacinamide is another popular ingredient that can help even out skin tone and support the skin's protective barrier, enhancing the benefits of peptides.

Some people also use exfoliating acids, like alpha hydroxy acids (AHAs), to remove dead cells on the surface. This might help peptides penetrate better. However, it is wise not to overdo exfoliation, as too much can irritate the skin. Balance is key.

10. Professional Treatments with Peptides

Aside from at-home products, there are professional treatments that use peptides, sometimes in conjunction with facial procedures. For instance, an esthetician might apply a peptide-rich serum during a session that involves micro-needling, which creates tiny channels in the skin to boost absorption. Or a specialist might combine peptides with light therapy or ultrasound treatments to help them sink in deeper. These approaches can be more intense than simply applying a cream at home.

While these professional methods can give a quick boost, they are not a permanent solution. Skin continues to change over time, and peptides must be used regularly to keep seeing benefits. Also, any procedure that disturbs the surface of the skin carries risks, like redness or infection if not done correctly. Always check the qualifications of anyone performing advanced skin treatments.

---

11. Safety and Side Effects

Generally, peptides in skin care are considered safe for most individuals. They rarely cause major side effects, but people with very sensitive skin might experience minor irritation. This could show up as redness, itching, or a slight rash. If this happens, it might be due to another ingredient in the product, such as fragrance, preservatives, or carriers. Doing a patch test before using a new peptide product on your face can help you catch issues early.

If you have a medical skin condition, it is wise to ask a dermatologist or other qualified professional before trying new products. While peptides are generally mild, you want to be certain there are no interactions with any treatments you are already using.

---

12. Do-It-Yourself vs. Store-Bought

Some people like to experiment with homemade skin care. Making a stable peptide product at home is very hard because peptides can break down if not stored correctly. Also, measuring the right concentration is tricky without proper tools. It is usually safer and more effective to buy products from brands that have tested their formulas. Many brands invest in research or partner with labs to ensure that the peptides stay active and do what they claim.

If you do go the homemade route, be cautious about sourcing. A random peptide powder from an unknown supplier may not be pure or may contain contaminants. It is typically best to stick to reputable brands or talk with a skin professional who can give you options that have been tested.

13. The Science Gap

One challenge with peptide skin care is that much of the research is done by the brands themselves or by small labs that might have a connection to the company making the product. This does not necessarily mean the findings are false, but it can be harder to find large, independent studies that confirm the effects. Skin is also complex, so what works in a small experiment might not work for everyone in real life.

Still, many dermatologists and consumers see benefits from peptide products, suggesting that at least some of the claims hold true. The best approach is to treat peptides as part of an overall routine. They can help encourage certain processes, but they are not a cure-all. Good skin care also involves sunscreen, gentle cleansing, balanced nutrition, and perhaps professional guidance if you have specific concerns.

---

14. Peptides vs. Other Active Ingredients

Skin care is full of active ingredients like retinoids, alpha hydroxy acids, and vitamin C. Each of these works in different ways. Retinoids boost cell turnover and support collagen, while AHAs remove old cells from the surface. Vitamin C helps with brightening and collagen. Peptides stand out for their ability to mimic or trigger signals in the skin without the stronger side effects that can come from retinoids or acids.

However, retinoids and acids have a longer track record and more extensive studies behind them. Peptides are still a growing field. That said, many people like peptides because they can be gentler. They may cause less flaking or redness compared to some other ingredients. For those with sensitive or very dry skin, peptides can be a starting point, possibly combined with lower doses of stronger ingredients.

---

15. Caring for the Skin from the Inside

Even the most advanced peptide cream will have limited power if other parts of skin care are ignored. The skin needs a steady supply of proteins, vitamins, and healthy fats to maintain its barrier. Drinking enough fluids, eating nutrient-rich foods, and protecting the skin from severe sun exposure can all help. Peptides on the surface can be a good addition, but they are not a complete answer if there is a serious lack of nutrients in the body.

Lifestyle factors also matter. Frequent stress or a lack of rest might show up on the skin as dullness or breakouts. Smoking can reduce blood flow and break down collagen faster. Uncontrolled sun exposure is a big factor in wrinkles and spots. So while peptides may help manage some of these effects, a long-term plan for healthy living is key.

---

16. Examples of Skin Care Routines with Peptides

Here is a basic outline of how someone might fit a peptide serum into a daily skin care routine:

1. **Morning**:
   - Wash face with a gentle cleanser.
   - Apply a toner or essence if desired.
   - Use a peptide serum or lotion.
   - Follow up with a moisturizer containing sunscreen, or apply a separate sunscreen.
2. **Evening**:
   - Remove makeup and cleanse the face.
   - Use a light exfoliant if recommended (but not every night).
   - Apply a peptide product, possibly along with other active ingredients like niacinamide or a mild retinoid.
   - Finish with a richer moisturizer if skin tends to be dry.

This routine is just an example, and people may choose different orders or skip certain steps. The main idea is to place peptide products before thicker creams so they can reach the skin effectively. Sunscreen is a must during the day to protect the skin and help maintain any benefits gained from peptides.

17. Professional Guidance

If you want to address significant skin concerns, it can be helpful to see a dermatologist. They can advise on whether peptides are right for your situation and suggest other treatments. In some cases, you might benefit more from prescription-strength retinoids, in-office procedures, or medical guidance for conditions like acne, eczema, or rosacea. Peptide products are generally mild and can fit into many routines, but serious or persistent issues often require medical care.

Dermatologists can also point you to clinical data on certain peptide ingredients. They might know which product lines have better backing or stability testing. Furthermore, they can help you set realistic expectations. While peptide-based products can be part of a good skin plan, results often take consistent use and will not be as dramatic as medical treatments like lasers or chemical peels.

---

18. Environmental Factors

The environment affects how well skin care products work. If you live in a very dry or cold area, your skin might lose moisture faster. This can reduce the benefits of peptides unless you also use a strong moisturizer or humidifier. In a hot, humid climate, you might sweat more, which can affect how products stay on the skin. Pollution and other factors can also impact skin health, so it is smart to tailor your routine to your local environment.

Peptides themselves do not offer protection from pollution or sun damage. However, some newer formulas attempt to pair peptides with antioxidants that help neutralize pollutants. Still, blocking or removing pollutants from the skin typically requires washing at the end of the day, using protective products, and staying aware of environmental conditions.

---

19. Trends in Peptide Skin Care

The peptide skin care market has grown quickly. Consumers can find all sorts of claims, from basic moisturizing creams that "contain peptides" to specialized serums that list specific peptide complexes. As with any trend, it is wise to be cautious. A product that puts "peptides" on the label might have only a tiny amount, or the peptides might not be stable. Reading reviews, asking dermatologists, and looking for brand transparency can help.

Some brands also highlight "bio-mimetic" peptides, meaning peptides that mimic natural signals in the skin. This is a promising approach, as it suggests the product is designed to communicate with cells the way the body does on its own. However, the quality and concentration still matter. Peptides need to be properly formulated and combined with the right ingredients. If a product does not share its peptide concentrations or rely on any studies, consumers should be careful with high expectations.

---

20. The Bottom Line on Peptides in Skin Care

Peptides are one of many tools in modern skin care. They can send helpful signals to skin cells, assist with collagen and elastin maintenance, or help keep the skin barrier in better shape. Some peptides come paired with metals or other additives to further support the skin's normal repair processes. When used regularly and combined with good habits like daily sun protection, a balanced diet, and gentle cleansing, peptides can be a valuable part of a skin care plan.

Still, it is important to remember that no single ingredient can do everything. The science behind peptides in skin care shows promise, but each individual's skin is different. If you are thinking of trying a peptide product, look for brands that provide clear information, stable packaging, and realistic claims. Even the most advanced peptide needs time to show noticeable effects, and long-term results will also depend on how well you care for your skin overall.

Peptides can help give your skin extra support, but they are not the only factor. Keep a balanced approach by combining peptide products with other helpful ingredients and healthy habits. In the following chapters, we will look at more ways peptides can be used, including how they might help in hair and nail health, and what role they might play in broader wellness practices. By seeing the full range of peptide uses, you can make informed choices about whether they fit your specific needs.

Chapter 7: Peptides and Signs of Aging

As people grow older, changes take place in many parts of the body. These changes can affect how someone looks and feels. Scientists have discovered that some of these changes are linked to shifts in important proteins and signals, many of which involve peptides. In this chapter, we will look at how aging can show up in skin, muscles, and other areas, and how peptides may help manage or slow down certain signs that come with age.

---

1. What Happens as We Age?

Aging is a natural process that affects every person. Over the years, cells in the body slowly lose some of their ability to grow and repair. This might result in less collagen in the skin, slower healing, and reduced flexibility in joints. Muscles can also get weaker, and the immune system may not respond as quickly. These gradual changes can make older adults more likely to feel tired or experience certain health concerns.

One important part of aging happens at the microscopic level. Each cell in the body has DNA and various proteins that run daily activities. Over time, DNA can accumulate damage, and the quality of protein production may not be as high. This leads to small errors that add up. The body does have ways to correct these errors or remove damaged cells, but these repairs are not perfect. Eventually, more and more cells may show signs of wear and tear.

Many proteins in our body need the help of peptides to do their work, or they are regulated by peptide signals. That is why researchers are studying how shifting levels of peptides might be tied to certain aging issues, such as weaker muscles or skin that does not bounce back as quickly. If we understand these signals, we can look for ways to support or restore them.

---

2. Collagen and Elastin: Peptide Connections

When people talk about aging, they often focus on changes in the skin. One main reason skin becomes thinner or less firm is the drop in collagen and elastin in the dermis. Collagen is like scaffolding for skin, while elastin helps it move and then return to its original shape. As we grow older, enzymes called collagenases and elastases can break down these proteins faster than the body replaces them.

Peptide-based products may help support collagen or elastin in a few ways. First, certain signal peptides can send messages to skin cells, asking them to make more collagen or other structural proteins. Second, some peptides can block the enzymes that destroy collagen and elastin. If the breakdown slows down, it might help skin maintain a bit more strength and elasticity.

That does not mean peptide products erase all signs of age, but they may be part of a plan to keep skin looking and feeling healthier. These peptides are added to skin creams, serums, or other topical formulas in the hope that they can pass through the skin barrier and reach the cells that produce collagen. Because people's skin varies widely, results can also vary. Still, the idea of using peptides to help slow collagen breakdown is a major reason they appear in many skin care lines for mature or photo-damaged skin.

---

3. Muscle Tone and Strength

Apart from skin changes, older adults also notice shifts in muscle mass and strength. This can be due to lower levels of growth-related signals that tell muscles to repair and build new fibers. Muscle tissues depend on proteins like actin and myosin to expand and contract. Peptide signals can support processes that help replace damaged muscle proteins.

Some peptides in the body help regulate the release of growth factors or hormones that help maintain muscle. When these levels drop, people may see a faster reduction in muscle mass, a process called sarcopenia. Researchers wonder if they can develop peptide-based therapies or supplements to slow or reduce this muscle decline. For instance, certain peptides might tell muscle cells to make more contractile proteins or better handle the nutrients needed for repair.

Additionally, there is interest in peptides that could help shorten muscle recovery time after exercise, especially for older folks who want to stay active. However, many of these approaches remain under study, and experts stress that physical activity, proper nutrition, and enough rest are also crucial for maintaining muscle mass over time.

---

4. Bone and Joint Health

Bones can weaken with age, leading to conditions like osteoporosis. Joints may also wear down, causing stiffness or discomfort. One factor behind these changes is that the body's production of structural proteins in bones and cartilage does not keep up with what is lost. This means bones and cartilage can gradually thin or become more fragile.

Peptides may be able to help maintain healthier bones by:

1. **Signaling Bone Growth**: Certain peptides may direct cells called osteoblasts to form fresh bone or reduce the activity of osteoclasts that break bone down.
2. **Supporting Cartilage**: Similar signals might encourage chondrocytes (cartilage-producing cells) to keep making the materials needed for flexible joints.

While the research here is still early, it opens the possibility that peptide-based treatments could team up with minerals like calcium and phosphorus to keep bones strong. Many older adults already rely on supplements like vitamin D or calcium to help bone health. Peptides might become part of that plan if future studies confirm their usefulness.

---

5. Immune System Changes

As a person ages, their immune system can become less responsive. This can mean slower recovery from infections or a higher risk of getting sick. Peptides play a major role in immune signals. For example, small messenger peptides can call certain immune cells to the site of an infection or injury. If these signals are no longer working well, the immune system might not react quickly or effectively enough.

Some peptide-based approaches aim to boost the immune response in older adults. One idea is to help immune cells recognize threats more effectively. Another is to manage chronic swelling, which can become more common with age and might increase the risk of health problems. By guiding the body's immune signals, peptides might offer a way to keep the immune system better balanced.

Balancing the immune system is tricky. You do not want it too weak, but you also do not want it in a constantly overactive state, which can harm tissues. Because of this, each new peptide therapy must be tested carefully to confirm that it keeps the immune response in a healthy range.

---

6. Cognitive Aspects and Brain Health

While getting older, many people worry about memory and other brain functions. There are many factors involved in changes to the brain, including blood flow, buildup of certain proteins, and the way cells talk to each other. Some peptides function as neurotransmitters or neuromodulators, which means they pass or modify signals between nerve cells.

If the brain's peptide balance is off, it might add to memory loss or changes in focus. Studies in labs are looking at whether peptide-based molecules can help nerve cells stay healthy for a longer time. Some peptides may help reduce the buildup of unwanted proteins in the brain, while others might help nerve cells form better connections. However, delivering peptides across the blood-brain barrier is not easy, so this is still a work in progress.

Beyond direct brain effects, there is also a link between general health and cognitive function. For example, high blood pressure or poor blood sugar control can harm brain cells. Because some peptides assist in regulating blood pressure or metabolism, they may indirectly support better brain function by helping keep blood flow and sugar levels balanced.

---

7. Metabolic Balance and Weight

As people age, they may notice that it is easier to gain weight and harder to lose it. This can happen for several reasons, such as slower metabolism, changes in activity level, and hormone fluctuations. Peptides are key players in how the body uses and stores energy. Certain peptide hormones control appetite, how quickly we feel full, and how the body processes sugars and fats.

If these peptide signals become less effective, a person may eat more than their body needs or have trouble managing blood sugar. Scientists have been studying peptide-based treatments to manage weight in some adults. For example, peptides that mimic hormones that reduce hunger can help people feel full sooner. Others may help the body manage sugar better, which can also affect weight.

While these treatments show promise, they are not a quick fix. Lifestyle choices—like balanced eating, moderate exercise, and enough sleep—remain the main ways to keep a stable weight. Peptides might be part of a bigger plan for certain people who struggle with weight changes linked to age or medical conditions.

---

8. Skin Appearance and Wrinkles

One of the most noticeable signs of aging appears on the skin's surface: wrinkles, fine lines, and dryness. The skin also can become more delicate and bruise more easily. A main driver of these changes is less collagen, but there are also changes in how the skin holds moisture. Natural oils may not be produced at the same rate, leading to dryness.

Peptides in anti-aging products aim to:

1. **Stimulate New Collagen**: Signal peptides can support the creation of new collagen, slowing the deepening of lines.
2. **Strengthen the Barrier**: Some peptide formulas help the outer layer of the skin stay hydrated. A more solid barrier can keep water in and harmful factors out.

3. **Soothe the Look of Wrinkles**: Neurotransmitter-inhibiting peptides might help soften facial expressions slightly, though these effects are usually milder than procedures in a clinic.

Even though peptides cannot remove all wrinkles, they might reduce some visible signs if used consistently. Sunscreen is also crucial. Sun damage is one of the biggest causes of visible aging in the skin, so protecting against UV rays can keep the positive effects of peptides from being undone.

9. Hormonal Changes

For many people, hormonal changes are a key part of aging, especially in mid-life years. Shifts in hormones can affect mood, metabolism, bone density, and more. Some of these hormones are made from larger proteins, but small peptides often act as signals within these hormone pathways. That is why there has been interest in using or studying certain peptides to support hormone balance.

For instance, in some cases, doctors might prescribe peptide-based medicines that signal the release of hormones involved in regulating sleep or reproduction. However, these therapies must be used carefully under medical guidance. Hormones are powerful, and changing them can have major side effects. Still, the possibility of using peptide signals to smooth out the hormone-related parts of aging is a focus for many researchers.

10. The Role of Antioxidant Peptides

With age, cells can experience oxidative stress, which happens when harmful molecules called free radicals build up. Antioxidants can help neutralize these free radicals before they cause damage. While most people think of vitamins and plant compounds as antioxidants, some peptides have antioxidant properties too.

Antioxidant peptides can come from food sources, such as certain protein-rich meals that get broken down into smaller chains. Researchers are also looking for ways to make or boost these peptides in the body to reduce oxidative damage that contributes to aging. Still, one should remember that diet, exercise, and avoiding too much sun exposure are also key ways to limit oxidative stress. A balanced approach can be more effective than relying on one peptide solution alone.

11. Sleep and Recovery

Getting enough good-quality sleep is important for people of any age, but older adults can experience shifts in sleep patterns. Some find it harder to fall asleep or stay asleep. Peptides in the body can help regulate sleep-wake cycles. For example, certain peptides that act as hormones are released at night to help the body rest and repair.

When the body rests, it puts more energy into fixing tissues, clearing out waste from cells, and recharging the immune system. If sleep is disrupted, these processes may suffer, possibly speeding up some signs of aging. Researchers are exploring whether certain peptide treatments could encourage better sleep. A more natural sleep rhythm might allow the body to handle repair tasks, which could show up as improvements in mood, energy, and overall well-being.

12. Supporting Healthy Aging Through Peptides

Healthy aging is about more than just looking younger. Many experts focus on "healthspan," which is how long a person stays active and in good health, rather than just lifespan. Peptides might support healthy aging in several ways:

1. **Backing Up Natural Repair**: By sending signals for growth or regeneration, peptides might help tissues cope with daily wear.
2. **Helping Metabolic Balance**: Certain peptide-based therapies or supplements may assist the body in handling sugars and fats.
3. **Assisting Immune Function**: Peptides that guide the immune system could keep it from becoming sluggish or overactive.
4. **Protecting Cells**: Some peptides act as antioxidants or reduce swelling, possibly easing the stress on cells.

These potential benefits do not mean peptides are a magic solution. A balanced diet, exercise, and regular health checkups are still very important. However, when used correctly, peptides may add a helpful layer of support.

---

13. Controlling Skin Tone and Brightness

Another change people notice as they get older is an uneven skin tone or dark spots that may appear after years of sun exposure. While these spots can show up at any age, they are more common in older adults. Melanin is the pigment that decides skin color, and it can collect in certain areas to cause patches or spots.

Some peptides can interfere with the enzymes that produce melanin. A few cosmetic products include these peptides to make the skin look more even or bright. The goal is not to bleach the skin, but to keep melanin from building up too much in certain areas. Combined with sunscreen, these products might help reduce the look of age spots over time.

---

14. Peptides in Alternative Treatments

In some alternative health circles, people talk about peptides as if they can do almost anything. They might use terms like "anti-aging peptide injections" or "peptide rejuvenation." While there is real science behind certain peptide therapies, a lot of these claims can be exaggerated, especially if there is no regulation or if the sources are not reliable. Some products are sold online without proper testing, which can be dangerous.

If you are thinking about any kind of peptide injection or supplement, it is important to get advice from a qualified healthcare provider. This is especially true for older adults who may be on other medications. Mixing peptides of unknown origin with prescription drugs or over-the-counter items can cause problems. A legitimate health provider will likely suggest a recognized product with a history of safety data.

---

15. Research and Clinical Trials

Ongoing research is looking at how peptides might help with specific parts of aging. For instance, some labs are testing if peptides can improve muscle mass in older people who do not respond well to exercise alone. Others are checking if peptide-based lotions can target deep wrinkles better than standard creams. Some trials also look at how peptides might reduce chronic swelling linked to age-related conditions.

The results of these studies will help confirm which peptides work best, how often they should be used, and for whom. If a certain peptide works wonders in a lab test but breaks down too quickly in the human body, it might not become a real therapy unless researchers find a way to stabilize it. Likewise, a peptide that works in younger adults might not behave the same way in older adults with different hormone levels or different metabolism.

---

16. Lifestyle Factors That Affect Peptide Action

Even with the best peptide therapy, lifestyle matters a lot. Peptides do not work in a vacuum. If someone is not getting enough protein in their diet, the body might lack the building blocks needed to make key peptides or other important molecules. If they rarely move or exercise, their muscles and bones will not get the signals they need to stay strong.

In addition, high levels of stress can release hormones that interfere with healthy cell function. Stress over a long period can speed up some markers of aging. While peptides might help in some ways, a person's overall stress level, sleep pattern, and daily routines all play a part. This is why many health experts say that any peptide therapy is best used alongside overall healthy habits.

---

17. Peptide Supplements vs. Medical Peptide Therapies

Not all peptides for aging are sold as medicines. Some come in the form of dietary supplements. These might contain collagen peptides or other chains claimed to support skin, joints, or digestion. These supplements can be found in powders, pills, or liquid forms. However, the quality and absorption of these supplements can differ. Some people report improvements in skin elasticity or joint comfort, but scientific data on how well they work can vary.

Medical peptide therapies, on the other hand, require a prescription and have been tested more thoroughly. They might come as injections or specialized formulations, often for managing a specific issue, like very poor muscle mass or a serious hormone imbalance. These treatments aim to deliver a carefully measured amount of a peptide known to have certain effects in the body.

In either case, it is wise to check for reputable brands, read labels, and talk to a healthcare professional. Older adults, especially, should be sure that supplements do not conflict with any prescriptions or other health conditions.

18. Skin Procedures and Peptides

Some cosmetic treatments in clinics include peptides for aging skin. For instance, micro-needling might be followed by applying a peptide solution to the treated area. Because micro-needling creates tiny channels in the skin, it might help the peptide penetrate more effectively. Another approach might be laser therapy that prepares the skin to better receive topical peptides.

These treatments can be more costly and not all have the same amount of scientific backing. If you are looking into such procedures, consider asking about the type of peptides used, the potential risks, and whether the clinic has data to support their method. While certain techniques show promise, results can depend on the skill of the provider and the individual's skin condition.

19. Long-Term Outlook

As science learns more about how aging works, it becomes clearer that it involves many moving parts. Peptides are just one aspect of the body's communications system. They might help reduce or slow certain signs, such as decreased collagen or muscle mass, but they cannot undo all the effects of time. The best results often come from combining multiple methods: healthy eating, staying active, managing stress, and using well-researched medical or cosmetic options if needed.

The future of peptide research for aging looks bright. We can expect more targeted peptides that address specific tissues or signals in the body. Delivery methods may improve, allowing peptides to stay active longer or reach deeper layers of the skin. Yet, it remains important to remember that the human body is complex, and there is no single ingredient that solves everything. With realistic expectations, peptides can be part of a thoughtful approach to aging that supports both appearance and health.

20. Key Points on Peptides and Aging

1. **Skin Firmness**: Peptides can support collagen and elastin, helping keep skin smoother for longer.
2. **Muscle Support**: Some peptides may encourage muscle repair, but exercise and nutrition are still vital.
3. **Bone Health**: Early findings suggest that peptides might help maintain bone density, in addition to minerals and vitamins.
4. **Immune Balance**: Peptides guide immune cells, helping keep the body defended without overreacting.
5. **Safe Use**: Always seek expert guidance for peptide injections or supplements, especially in older adulthood.
6. **Realistic Expectations**: Peptides are not a magical fix. They are one piece in a bigger plan that includes lifestyle choices.

Aging is natural, and while it can bring challenges, it can also be managed in ways that support overall well-being. Peptides offer exciting possibilities, but they work best when paired with basic healthy habits and regular medical checkups. By learning how these small chains of amino acids affect our cells and tissues, we may find new avenues to stay active and feel good as we grow older.

Chapter 8: Peptides for Hair and Nail Health

Healthy hair and strong nails can be signs of good overall well-being. But hair and nails can face problems like breakage, dryness, or slow growth. Some of these issues can happen with normal changes over time, but they can also come from poor nutrition, harsh styling methods, or medical conditions. In this chapter, we will see how peptides might help with hair and nail health, whether through supportive products, better nutrition, or targeted treatments.

---

1. Why Hair and Nails Matter

Hair and nails serve practical functions. Hair can help protect the scalp from sunburn, while nails shield the delicate tips of fingers and toes. But they also have a social or personal side—people often style their hair or maintain their nails for appearances or self-confidence.

When hair begins to thin or nails start to chip often, it can hint at internal changes. Nutrient deficiencies, hormone shifts, or damage from the environment can all show up in hair and nails. That is why many professionals look at hair and nail quality as part of a bigger health picture.

---

2. Structure of Hair and Nails

Hair fibers and nails are both made of a protein called keratin. Keratin is formed when specialized cells create large amounts of this protein and then die off, leaving a strong, protective layer. Keratin is also present in animal hooves and horns, showing how tough it can be.

1. **Hair:**
   - The visible part is the hair shaft, made mostly of keratin in layers.
   - Below the surface is the hair follicle, which has living cells that divide and grow, pushing the shaft upward.
   - Blood vessels deliver nutrients to the follicle, helping the hair grow.
2. **Nails:**

- The nail plate is the hard visible part.
- The nail matrix under the skin is where new nail cells form.
- As these cells make keratin, they get pushed out, forming the plate that you see.

Since hair and nails are largely made of proteins, it makes sense that peptides, which are amino-acid chains, could play a role in how they grow or remain strong.

---

3. How Peptides Can Support Hair

Peptides may assist hair health in a few ways:

1. **Scalp Environment**: Some peptides can soothe or support the scalp, helping skin cells there. A healthier scalp can encourage stronger hair growth.
2. **Keratin Production**: Certain peptides might guide cells in the hair follicle to ramp up keratin production or maintain the quality of the hair shaft.
3. **Blood Flow**: Some topical products claim they include peptides that widen blood vessels in the scalp, boosting the supply of nutrients to the follicles.

Because hair growth is a slow process, it can take time to see if peptide products make a difference. Also, each person's hair health depends on genetics, hormones, and overall wellness. Still, peptides are often included in shampoos, conditioners, and leave-in treatments with the idea that they can reinforce the hair shaft or help keep the follicle healthier.

---

4. Peptides for Thinning Hair

Thinning hair is common among adults, especially as they grow older. Sometimes, it is related to hormones like DHT (dihydrotestosterone), which can make hair follicles shrink. In other cases, thinning comes from stress, low protein intake, or certain medical conditions.

Peptide products for thinning hair often focus on:

- **Strengthening Roots**: They may try to block signals that lead to shrinking follicles.
- **Improving Cell Signaling**: Peptides might encourage growth factors that extend the active growth phase of the hair cycle.
- **Reducing Irritation**: If swelling in the scalp contributes to thinning, a soothing peptide might help keep the follicles in a better environment.

It is important to note that severe hair loss might need medical treatments or prescription medications, and not all hair thinning can be reversed by peptides. However, some individuals find that peptide-enriched formulas, used over many months, help their hair look fuller or more robust.

---

5. Peptides and Hair Care Products

When you visit a beauty store, you might see hair care lines featuring "peptide technology." They might list ingredients like "keratin peptides," "collagen peptides," or "copper peptide complexes." The idea behind these products is that when applied to the hair shaft or scalp, the peptides can provide support or signals that reduce breakage or dryness.

- **Keratin Peptides**: These can be small pieces of keratin that might fill in damaged spots in the hair shaft, somewhat like patching up holes.
- **Collagen Peptides**: Sometimes added to conditioner or mask formulas for a smoothing effect. They may help hair feel softer, although collagen peptides primarily focus on skin and structural support.
- **Copper Peptide Formulas**: Some claim to boost scalp health by increasing blood flow or encouraging better cell function at the root.

These products vary in quality. Some contain enough of the active peptides to have an effect, while others might just use the word "peptide" for marketing. It is helpful to check reviews or talk to hair professionals before investing in expensive treatments. Also, keep in mind that any topical product needs consistent use over time.

6. Diet, Protein, and Hair Growth

Because hair is mostly protein, the body needs a steady supply of amino acids from food. If the diet does not include enough protein, or if the body lacks certain vitamins or minerals, hair may become brittle or grow more slowly. Some people choose to take collagen or amino acid supplements, hoping this will help hair growth. Others rely on a balanced diet rich in proteins like eggs, beans, or lean meats.

Peptides in supplements might be broken down into amino acids once they are in the digestive system. The body can then reassemble these amino acids into the proteins it needs. Whether this directly helps hair or nails can depend on many factors, including overall nutrition and health status. Some studies suggest that collagen peptides can improve hair thickness or reduce breakage, but results differ. If a person is already well-fed and healthy, extra peptides might not make a huge difference. On the other hand, if someone is low in protein, it might help.

7. Stress and Hair Loss

Stress can cause certain types of hair shedding. When under a lot of stress, the body might redirect resources away from hair growth. This can push hair follicles into a resting phase, leading to more shedding a few months later. While peptides can be part of scalp care, handling stress in other ways—like relaxation techniques or good sleep—remains vital.

Some new research looks at whether small peptides can help buffer the effects of stress hormones on hair follicles. However, this is still a growing area of study. It shows that many things can affect hair, and peptides are just one piece of the puzzle.

8. Nail Growth and Strength

Nails also rely on keratin. Factors that affect nails include diet, daily activities, exposure to chemicals or water, and certain diseases. When nails get weak, they might split or peel easily. Like hair, nails need a steady flow of proteins and nutrients to stay healthy.

Peptides for nail health can:

1. **Deliver Amino Acids**: Some products include hydrolyzed keratin peptides in nail creams or cuticle oils, aiming to nourish the nail plate or surrounding skin.
2. **Improve Moisture Balance**: If the nail or cuticle is too dry, it can crack. Peptides that help hold moisture might keep the nail area more flexible.
3. **Encourage Better Cell Production**: Signal peptides might prompt the nail matrix cells to produce stronger keratin.

Again, real-world results vary, and nails grow slowly—around three millimeters a month for fingernails, even slower for toenails. So it can take a while to see improvements.

---

9. Common Peptides for Hair and Nail Products

Below are some peptides you might find in hair and nail care labels:

1. **Keratin Hydrolysates**: These are partly broken-down keratin molecules that can be small enough to attach to hair or nail surfaces.
2. **Collagen Peptides**: They may strengthen the tissue surrounding the nails and hair follicles.
3. **Copper Peptides**: Often included to support the scalp or nail bed by helping with blood flow and cell signals.
4. **Polypeptide Complexes**: Some brands blend different amino acid chains, each aiming for a specific effect.

Since it is difficult to prove how well each type works, especially when combined, reading unbiased reviews or consulting a hair or nail specialist can help. Look for products that come from well-known manufacturers that invest in research rather than those making grand claims with little evidence.

10. Professional Treatments and Peptide Boosters

Hair salons and nail salons sometimes offer special treatments that claim to use peptide technology. In a hair salon, for example, a stylist might apply a concentrated peptide mask after coloring or bleaching to help reduce breakage. Nail salons might have peptide-based strengthening formulas applied like polish.

These treatments can be more potent than store-bought products, but they also cost more. If done correctly, they may repair damaged hair cuticles or weak nails for a while. However, the effects might wear off if you return to harsh styling methods or do not keep up with proper care at home.

Other professional approaches might include micro-needling on the scalp along with a peptide serum to help with hair thinning. As with any procedure, it is wise to talk about risks, costs, and realistic outcomes before proceeding. Such treatments might help some people, but they are not guaranteed to work for everyone.

---

11. Differences in Hair and Nail Growth Cycles

Hair grows in cycles. There is an active phase (anagen), a transition phase (catagen), and a resting phase (telogen). After the resting phase, the hair falls out, and a new one starts to grow. This process can be influenced by hormones, nutrients, and overall health. In thinning hair, the active phase might get shorter, or more follicles might enter the resting phase. Peptides might aim to extend the active phase or reduce the resting phase, though the success depends on many factors.

Nail growth is steadier, with the nail matrix continuously creating new cells. The speed of growth can be influenced by age, blood circulation, and overall health. If nails get insufficient nutrients, they might grow more slowly or with ridges. While peptides cannot directly speed up the underlying biology of cell division beyond normal limits, they can help ensure that cells have the building blocks they need.

---

12. Hormonal Connections

Hormones play a big role in hair and nail growth. Changes in hormones can cause sudden hair loss or changes in nail texture. For example, after pregnancy or during menopause, women can experience a shift in hair thickness or nail quality. Men can also notice changes linked to hormone levels over time.

Peptide-based products usually work outside the hormone system, though some might slightly adjust signals in the scalp or nail bed. They are not likely to fix major hormone-driven issues on their own, but they might help reduce some of the visible effects. A doctor might recommend a hormone test or other treatments if hair loss or brittle nails seem to be tied to major hormone imbalances.

---

13. Avoiding Damage

While peptides can help, they will be less effective if hair or nails face constant harm. For hair, repeated bleaching, tight hairstyles that pull on follicles, or constant heat styling can cause breakage. For nails, habits like biting, picking, or using nails as tools can lead to splits. Frequent exposure to water or harsh chemicals (like strong cleaning products) can weaken nails as well.

Here are ways to protect hair and nails:

1. **Use Gentle Products**: Choose milder shampoos and conditioners or soaps that do not strip away natural oils.
2. **Limit Heat**: Frequent use of hot styling tools can dry out hair. Aim for lower temperatures or use protective sprays.
3. **Shield Nails**: Wear gloves when cleaning or washing dishes.
4. **Manage Stress**: Stress can weaken hair and nails from the inside.
5. **Eat Balanced Meals**: Provide your body with nutrients, including enough protein, vitamins, and minerals.

With less daily harm, peptides in hair or nail care products can do more good.

14. Nail and Hair Supplements

Many stores sell supplements labeled for hair and nail growth. They might include vitamins (like biotin), minerals (like zinc and iron), and sometimes collagen or other peptide powders. People often wonder if these help. Biotin, for instance, is a B vitamin important for protein building, but unless you have a deficiency, extra biotin might not dramatically change hair or nails.

That said, if someone's hair or nails are weak due to low intake of protein or certain nutrients, a supplement might help fill the gap. Some supplements have blends of amino acids or collagen peptides that could offer building blocks for keratin. Results can take months to appear, as hair and nail growth is slow. If your diet is already rich in the needed nutrients, you might not see much difference. Always check with a healthcare provider before adding new supplements, especially if you have any health conditions.

---

15. Popular Myths

There are several myths about hair and nails:

1. **Trimming Makes Them Grow Faster**: Trimming hair or nails regularly can help remove split ends or ragged edges, but it does not speed up their growth from the root.
2. **All Protein Treatments Are the Same**: Not every "protein" or "peptide" product is equally effective. Some might only coat the surface, while others can bond more deeply.
3. **Overnight Miracles**: Building stronger hair or nails takes time. Any product claiming instant, permanent changes is likely just masking problems temporarily.

Peptides can help support hair and nail health, but they follow the body's pace of growth. Patience and a healthy routine often bring the best results.

---

16. The Role of the Scalp and Cuticles

For hair, the scalp environment is critical. If the scalp is overly oily, dry, or filled with buildup, follicles might struggle. Peptides in scalp serums can target dryness or help balance oil production. For nails, the cuticle area is where new nail cells get some protection. Products that include peptides may soften or moisturize the cuticle, helping the new cells to grow in a stronger way. Keeping these regions clean and well cared for supports healthy growth.

17. Combining Peptides with Other Helpful Ingredients

Many hair and nail products mix peptides with other beneficial components:

- **Hyaluronic Acid**: Retains moisture, which can reduce dryness in hair or nails.
- **Natural Oils**: Like argan or jojoba oils, which help seal the hair shaft and protect nails.
- **Plant Extracts**: Some extracts contain antioxidants that protect hair follicles or nail cells from harmful molecules.
- **Ceramides**: These are lipids that can help restore a damaged hair cuticle or fortify the nail barrier.

Peptides often work better as part of these formulas than by themselves, since hair and nails need multiple types of nourishment and protection.

18. Professional Advice

If you have serious hair loss, patchy bald spots, or very brittle nails, it might be time to see a professional. A dermatologist or trichologist (hair and scalp specialist) can check for underlying issues such as thyroid problems or nutrient deficiencies. They might suggest blood tests or examine the scalp more closely. You can also ask them about peptide-based solutions or other treatments that fit your condition.

Sometimes, hair or nail trouble is a sign of something else going on inside the body. When the core issue is treated, hair and nail quality can improve. Peptides can be a helpful add-on, but they are often not the main solution if a bigger health concern is at play.

19. Setting Expectations

Peptides can help hair look and feel stronger, and they may enhance nail quality. However, big changes usually need time. Hair grows only about one centimeter per month on average, and nails grow only a couple of millimeters per month. This means you might not notice significant differences for a few months of consistent use. If a product claims you will "wake up" with completely transformed hair or nails, that is not realistic.

It is also smart to look for subtle signs of improvement first—less breakage, a bit more shine, or fewer split ends in hair. For nails, maybe they peel less or do not chip as easily. Small steps add up, and a consistent routine is often better than using many different products briefly.

---

20. Conclusion: Peptides as Part of a Broader Strategy

Keeping hair and nails strong goes beyond a single ingredient. It includes a good diet, gentle grooming, protection from harsh chemicals or styling tools, and watching for underlying health issues. Peptides fit into this picture by offering support:

1. **Topical Application**: Shampoos, conditioners, serums, and nail creams with peptides can coat or strengthen the surface. Some are designed to soak in and help at a deeper level.
2. **Internal Support**: Collagen or other peptide supplements might provide amino acids to build better keratin, particularly if there is a shortage of dietary protein.
3. **Scalp and Nail Bed Care**: Peptides that calm swelling or boost circulation might give hair follicles or the nail matrix a healthier place to grow.

Results depend on each person's genetics, age, hormone balance, and environment. But for those looking to improve hair thickness or nail strength, peptides can be a valuable piece of the plan. Just keep in mind that everything from how often you wash your hair to what you eat at breakfast can play a role in how effective these products or supplements are.

Chapter 9: Peptides and Weight Management

People often think about body weight and how to keep it in a healthy range. Managing weight involves balancing the amount of energy taken in through food with the energy used during activity and normal bodily functions. Peptides have become a point of interest for those studying ways to assist this balance. Researchers have found certain peptide signals that tell us when we feel hungry or full, or that help the body handle sugars and fats. In this chapter, we will discuss how these peptides work, how they may support weight goals, and what limits or concerns come with their use.

---

1. The Basics of Body Weight Balance

The body gets energy from the foods we eat, mainly carbohydrates, fats, and proteins. When we eat more calories than we use, our bodies can store the extra as fat. When we use more energy than we eat, our bodies must burn stored fat or other tissues for fuel. Over time, changes in weight can happen when one side of this balance is out of line with the other.

While simple math suggests eating less or moving more can help with weight control, biology is more complicated. Many signals in the body influence how hungry we feel, how fast we burn energy, and where our bodies store fat. Some of these signals are peptides. These short chains of amino acids can move through the bloodstream or work in nearby areas to guide the body's decisions about food intake and storage.

---

2. Peptide Hormones for Appetite

Ghrelin

One well-known peptide connected to hunger is ghrelin. When the stomach is empty, ghrelin levels go up. The signal travels to the brain and triggers hunger feelings, causing us to look for food. Once we eat, ghrelin levels usually drop, and hunger fades. Some people have called ghrelin the "hunger hormone" because of its ability to encourage eating. If ghrelin signals stay high for too long, it might prompt overeating, which can add to weight gain.

Peptide YY (PYY)

After a meal, cells in the intestines release another peptide, known as PYY. It tells the brain that we have eaten, lowering the desire for more food. People with higher PYY levels might feel fuller sooner, which can help keep them from overdoing calories. Some research has checked whether raising PYY levels could help people control weight, but this must be done carefully to avoid problems like not getting enough nutrition or feeling sick.

Cholecystokinin (CCK)

This peptide hormone also goes up after eating, especially when fatty or protein-rich foods are digested. It slows down how fast the stomach empties, letting the brain catch up with signals of fullness. By lengthening the time food stays in the stomach, CCK can reduce the wish to eat more. It also helps release enzymes and bile to break down food. While CCK is not always called just a "peptide"—it is often called a "peptide hormone"—it still fits into the category of short amino-acid chains that have a direct effect on appetite and digestion.

---

3. Peptides that Affect Sugar Control

Blood sugar levels play a major role in weight. When blood sugar is stable, people often feel steady energy and fewer strong cravings. If blood sugar swings a lot, it can cause hunger spikes and lead to overeating. Certain peptides help manage how the body responds to sugar.

Glucagon-Like Peptide-1 (GLP-1)

GLP-1 is a peptide released in the gut after a meal. It encourages the pancreas to release insulin, which helps cells take in sugar from the blood. GLP-1 also slows stomach emptying and tells the brain that we are full. Because of these effects, drugs that mimic GLP-1 have become popular for people who have trouble with blood sugar control. Some of these drugs can also support weight management by keeping appetite in check.

Amylin

Amylin is a peptide made by the pancreas along with insulin. It helps control how fast food moves through the stomach and signals fullness. Some people who do not produce enough insulin might also have low amylin levels. Researchers wonder if amylin-like drugs could help people handle their blood sugar and appetite better. Certain treatments based on amylin are being tested or used in specific medical cases.

---

4. How Peptide Therapies for Weight Work

When a peptide therapy is used for weight, it often copies or boosts a natural peptide in the body. For example, a synthetic version of GLP-1 might last longer than the natural form, giving the person a more prolonged feeling of fullness. This can help them eat less and lose extra weight over time. Because peptides can be designed to aim at particular receptors in the body, they can have effects that are more targeted than some older drugs.

Many of these therapies involve injections, because peptides can be broken down in the stomach if taken by mouth. This can make peptide-based weight treatments more complex and costly than a pill. Researchers are looking into ways to deliver peptides differently, such as by nasal spray or protective capsules, but these methods are still being tested.

It is also important to note that no peptide therapy replaces a balanced approach to eating and activity. Even if a person uses a peptide drug that reduces hunger, they must still choose healthy foods and stay active. Peptides might lower harmful cravings or help control portion sizes, but the overall lifestyle still matters a lot.

---

5. Examples of Peptide-Based Weight Support

Several peptide-based drugs or research directions focus on weight control:

1. **GLP-1 Agonists**: Designed to act like GLP-1 but last longer in the body, these reduce hunger and help manage blood sugar.

2. **Dual or Triple Agonists**: Some new treatments combine the actions of more than one gut hormone, like GLP-1, GIP, and glucagon, hoping for a stronger effect on weight or sugar.
3. **Amylin Mimetics**: These copy the actions of amylin to slow stomach emptying and signal fullness.

These treatments often require a prescription and medical oversight because they can have side effects, such as feelings of nausea or issues if the dose is too high. They are usually intended for people with a medical need, such as those with certain metabolic conditions or a high risk of complications from extra weight.

---

6. Challenges and Side Effects

Peptides that help weight management can be powerful, but they may also come with challenges:

- **Nausea and Digestive Upset**: Many appetite-related peptides slow the rate at which the stomach empties. This can lead to queasiness or bloating.
- **Cost and Accessibility**: Peptide drugs can be expensive, and not all health plans cover them.
- **Need for Ongoing Use**: Some people find that once they stop a peptide therapy, their appetite returns to its old patterns. Without addressing other parts of life, weight might come back.
- **Individual Differences**: People respond differently to the same peptide therapy. What works for one person may not work as well for another.

These points mean that each person must talk with a doctor about whether peptide-based treatments fit their situation. It also means that relying only on peptides without healthy habits may not bring lasting improvements.

---

7. Dietary Peptides and Weight

Peptides do not only come as medicines. Some foods can break down into small peptides during digestion. Certain diets high in protein can lead to increased levels of peptides in the gut. These might help people feel fuller after meals. This is one reason why balanced protein intake can be helpful for some who want to manage weight.

For example, casein in dairy can produce small peptides when it is digested, which may reduce hunger. Soy proteins can also yield peptides that show potential for supporting healthy blood pressure or fullness. Research is ongoing, but many nutrition experts suggest including enough protein at each meal to help manage appetite, with or without special peptide formulas.

---

8. Fad Products and Caution

Because peptides are an active area of interest, some products are marketed online with claims to melt fat or erase cravings instantly. Buyers need to be careful. Not all products labeled with "peptides" are legitimate or safe. Some items could have unknown ingredients or may not have been tested well. Others might have very small amounts of peptides, so they have no real effect.

When looking at a peptide weight product, it is wise to:

1. **Check for Reputable Brands**: Products with good manufacturing standards are often safer.
2. **Ask a Professional**: A dietitian, doctor, or pharmacist can help figure out if a product is valid or risky.
3. **Read the Fine Print**: Be wary of big promises without proof. Real science usually shows modest benefits and notes possible side effects.

Peptide therapies, when properly tested and prescribed, can be valuable. However, "quick fix" options that skip medical guidance can be dangerous or simply not work.

---

9. Peptides and Metabolism

Aside from affecting hunger, certain peptides may influence how the body burns calories or stores fat. For instance, peptides related to growth factors can help maintain muscle, which in turn can raise the number of calories burned at rest. Other peptides might guide the release of energy from fat tissues.

Still, changes in metabolism from peptide interventions are often modest compared to the effects of exercise, muscle mass, and daily calorie intake. If a therapy can help a person keep muscle while losing fat, that can be helpful for their overall weight and fitness, but it does not mean they can ignore basic physical activities like walking or resistance training.

---

10. Combining Peptide Treatments with Other Approaches

For many people, the best outcomes come from combining methods. Peptide therapies might reduce hunger or aid sugar balance, but a healthy eating plan can improve nutrient intake and prevent big spikes in blood sugar. Physical activity increases energy usage, helps keep muscle, and improves mood. Sleep is also important, since poor rest can raise hunger hormones and make it harder to manage weight.

By aligning these factors—diet, exercise, sleep, and possibly peptide support—individuals can build a more lasting approach. A person who relies on a peptide alone might lose some weight at first but could find it hard to maintain if old habits remain. Peptides may give them the starting push, but regular habits keep them on track.

---

11. Future Research

Scientists keep studying peptide-based weight options. Some labs are looking at molecules that target more than one hunger or metabolic pathway at once. Others want to improve how peptides are delivered, maybe through pills that survive the stomach's acids. The hope is to find safe, effective treatments that do not cause too many side effects.

There is also interest in personalizing therapies. Since everyone's metabolism and genes differ, the same peptide might not work for each person. Doctors of the future might check a patient's hormone levels or genetic profile to pick the best peptide approach. Though it may be years away, this kind of tailored method could reduce trial and error.

12. Real-World Stories

Some people who have used peptide drugs for weight management share that they felt less urge to overeat, making it simpler to choose smaller portions or avoid snacks. Others mention that any weight they lost returned if they quit their medication without changing their meals or exercise routines. This shows that while peptides can be a helpful tool, they are not a permanent solution if a person reverts to the lifestyle that caused weight gain before.

Health professionals often point out that even moderate weight improvements can help lower risks like high blood pressure or joint stress. A small drop in weight can still bring real health benefits. Peptide therapies might make this process less daunting for those who struggle with constant hunger or sugar spikes.

---

13. Peptides for Specific Groups

While some peptide-based weight aids might be helpful, they are not for everyone. For instance, children, pregnant women, or people with certain medical conditions may need different considerations. A doctor might be extra cautious before prescribing a peptide for someone with heart disease or low blood pressure. Interactions with other medications must also be checked.

Even dietary peptides from high-protein foods need balance. Older individuals sometimes do well with slightly higher protein intake to maintain muscle and healthy weight, while those with kidney issues might need to watch protein amounts. The solution often depends on a person's overall health profile.

---

14. Emotional Side of Weight

Weight management can involve emotional challenges. Stress or sadness might lead people to eat even when not truly hungry. Peptides that manage physical hunger do not always address emotional or habitual eating patterns. Some people benefit from counseling or support groups that help them handle stress and get past unhelpful eating habits.

Peptide treatments can help reduce the physical signals that drive overeating, but the person may still need to work on mental and behavioral parts. This is where a therapist or a coach might assist, offering ways to cope with cravings that come from emotions instead of real hunger.

15. Quick Wins vs. Long-Term Changes

Some folks might be tempted to use peptides to see a fast drop in weight. While some changes might appear quickly, the real test is keeping the weight off. If a peptide only helps for a short time, weight can creep back up unless the person has changed how they eat and move.

Researchers often measure the success of a weight therapy by how many people keep the weight off for a year or two. The best results usually come from combining medical help with lifestyle changes that continue after the therapy ends. This is why many doctors stress forming healthy habits and not just depending on medication.

16. The Place of Peptides in a Healthy Life

Peptide approaches are part of a bigger puzzle. They might help control portions or balance blood sugar so that a person can focus on nutritious meals. They can help reduce constant hunger or big sugar dips. Still, people using these methods might do best if they also learn about healthy foods, ways to deal with stress, and exercises that fit their abilities.

A well-rounded routine might include:

- **Balanced Meals**: Lean proteins, whole grains, fruits, and vegetables.
- **Regular Activity**: Anything from daily walks to structured gym sessions.
- **Enough Sleep**: Aim for 7-9 hours a night, depending on age and personal needs.
- **Mindful Eating**: Notice hunger signals and try to eat slowly.
- **Medical Checkups**: Monitor important markers like blood pressure, cholesterol, and blood sugar.

Peptides can fit into this picture as an extra help, but they are rarely the only tool used.

17. Safety Testing

Medical peptides for weight are tested in controlled trials before approval. Researchers check if they truly aid weight management, how safe they are at different doses, and whether people develop new problems while on them. Studies also track if any benefits continue after stopping the therapy.

If a peptide drug makes it through these trials and gains approval from health authorities, it might still be monitored in the market. Doctors and patients can report any unusual effects, helping keep track of long-term safety. Sometimes, new warnings appear after more people use a drug. This monitoring process is an ongoing part of medical regulation.

18. Peptides and Active Lifestyles

Many people want to lose fat but maintain or grow muscle. Peptides that help balance appetite can be paired with exercise to encourage the body to burn more fat while keeping muscle. Consuming enough protein is also key, giving the body amino acids to repair muscle tissue after workouts.

Some individuals fear losing muscle if they cut calories too much. With a carefully structured plan, plus advice from a dietitian or trainer, they can try to shed excess fat while protecting lean mass. Peptides might assist by making it easier to stay on track with smaller meals, reducing the chance of overeating.

19. Reading Labels and Sources

If you shop for supplements that contain peptides to manage weight, remember:

- **Look for Third-Party Tests**: This can show a product has been checked for purity.

- **Check Ingredient Lists**: Sometimes "peptides" appear alongside many other active substances, making it hard to know which ingredient does what.
- **Avoid Overhyped Claims**: Terms like "burn fat instantly" or "no need to exercise" are red flags.

A health expert can offer better guidance on whether a product is safe and worth trying. In some cases, the simpler solution is just to eat a balanced, protein-rich diet and reduce junk food. Peptide supplements might not add much unless there is a known deficiency or a specific plan in place.

---

20. Final Thoughts on Peptides and Weight

Peptides can shape hunger signals, help manage blood sugar, and guide how the body uses energy. Some therapies based on peptides show promise for individuals who struggle to keep a healthy weight. However, these treatments are not a simple or universal fix. The body is complex, and real progress often requires addressing both the physical and behavioral sides of weight.

By learning how peptides function, a person can see if they might fit into their approach. For those with metabolic issues, peptide medicines supervised by a doctor can be a valuable tool. For others, focusing on a balanced lifestyle might be enough. In either case, peptides can be an extra option, but success often depends on combining them with overall healthy habits that last.

Chapter 10: Peptides in Athletic Performance

Athletes work hard to improve their endurance, strength, and recovery. They look for safe and effective methods to help them train and compete. While classic approaches like structured workouts, a balanced diet, and enough rest remain key, some athletes also explore peptides. Certain peptides might boost muscle repair, manage fatigue, or sharpen focus. Yet, this area can be controversial. Some peptides are not allowed in sports, and others require careful use under medical guidance. In this chapter, we will explore how peptides might help athletes, along with the concerns about fairness and safety.

---

1. Why Athletes Look at Peptides

Sports, especially at high levels, demand a lot from the body. Muscles experience wear and tear, and intense training can lead to micro-injuries that need healing. Endurance athletes push their heart, lungs, and energy systems to the limit. If peptides can help speed repair or increase stamina, that might give an athlete an edge.

Also, training can leave athletes sore or tired for days. If peptides can help them bounce back sooner, they can return to practice or competition faster. Some peptides might assist the body in using fats or sugars more efficiently. Others could help regulate inflammation so that tissues are not damaged by too much swelling after workouts.

However, performance improvements must be weighed against ethics, rules, and health. Many sports organizations have strict guidelines on which substances athletes can use. Substances that unfairly boost performance or pose health risks are often restricted.

---

2. Muscle Growth and Repair

Muscles adapt to exercise by making more proteins to handle heavier loads. This process depends on signals that tell muscle cells to create new fibers. Some peptides in the body help by activating growth pathways, especially after a hard workout. For instance, peptides linked to growth hormone or insulin-like growth factor (IGF-1) can encourage muscle tissue to repair faster and grow stronger.

Researchers have also investigated smaller peptides, sometimes called "growth factors," that may improve muscle fiber function. When the body repairs muscle, it breaks down old or damaged fibers and builds new ones. Peptides might speed up this process by guiding certain cells—like satellite cells in muscles—to divide and fuse with existing fibers.

Some athletes are curious about synthetic peptides that mimic these signals, thinking they might build muscle more quickly. But these same peptides might be on banned lists in many sports. Athletes must check if using them is allowed.

---

3. Endurance and Oxygen Delivery

Endurance depends on how well the body can deliver oxygen to muscles and how efficiently muscles use it. Proteins like hemoglobin carry oxygen in the blood, but certain peptides affect blood vessel opening or the production of new red blood cells. If a peptide can widen blood vessels (vasodilation), it might help with blood flow to muscles, reducing fatigue.

In high-altitude training or intense endurance sports, the body naturally increases substances like EPO (erythropoietin), which is a hormone that triggers red blood cell production. Synthetic versions of EPO are banned in most competitive sports. While EPO itself is larger than a short peptide, some smaller peptides can also play a part in signaling red blood cell production. Again, many of these are restricted by anti-doping agencies.

---

4. Injury Prevention and Joint Care

Athletes place stress on joints and connective tissues. Tissues like tendons and ligaments can tear or get inflamed if pushed too hard. Some peptides might help these tissues stay flexible and recover from minor damage. A healthy tendon or ligament can handle heavier training, potentially lowering injury risk.

Peptides that encourage collagen formation or reduce destructive enzymes in joint tissues might be used in certain treatments. Even if they do not directly enhance performance, they might help an athlete train more steadily by avoiding downtime. Some recovery treatments also include peptide-rich gels or injections aimed at quicker repair of muscle or tendon injuries. However, these methods must be done under qualified medical care to avoid complications.

5. Reducing Swelling and Pain

Hard training or competition causes minor tears in muscle fibers, leading to swelling and soreness. While some swelling is a normal step in healing, too much can delay recovery. Certain peptides can act on the body's immune system to keep swelling under control, helping athletes feel less discomfort. This might allow them to return to practice sooner and be more consistent with their workouts.

Yet, athletes should be mindful. If peptides reduce swelling too much, they might train or compete on an injury before it has fully healed. That could lead to worse damage. Balancing normal healing with the desire to push forward is always important. Coaches and sports medicine experts often say that some muscle soreness is a natural sign that you worked hard, and it should not always be blocked.

6. Mental Sharpness and Stress

High-level sports can bring mental stress. Athletes must maintain focus and manage pressure. While many factors shape mental state, some peptides and protein-based hormones can affect mood, alertness, or stress responses. For example, the body releases certain peptides during stress, which can affect how tense or calm a person feels.

There is talk of using peptides to help with calmness or mental clarity, but reliable evidence in athletic settings is limited. Also, doping rules might apply if a peptide changes alertness or provides an advantage. Many sports authorities are watchful for any substance that might influence mental or physical performance beyond normal training.

7. Approved Medical Uses vs. Athletic Use

Some peptides are approved for treating certain health conditions. For example, growth hormone treatments can be prescribed if someone's body does not make enough on its own. However, using these peptides for athletic advantage is typically not allowed by sports rules. A medication that is helpful for someone with a real hormone deficiency can be considered cheating in sports if used by a healthy athlete to gain more muscle or stamina.

Athletes who have medical conditions sometimes need special permission (a therapeutic use exemption) to use certain substances. They must prove that they truly need the treatment and are not trying to gain an unfair edge. The process can involve detailed medical tests and documentation.

8. Anti-Doping Rules

Groups like the World Anti-Doping Agency (WADA) keep lists of substances that athletes cannot use in competitions. Many peptides that raise growth hormone levels, increase red blood cell production, or change the body's signals in ways that give an advantage are on the banned list. If an athlete is found to have these substances in their system without a valid medical reason, they can face penalties such as suspension or being stripped of titles.

Tests can detect certain peptides, though some are tricky to trace. Researchers keep developing new tests to catch banned peptide use. Because of the risk of detection and punishment, athletes must be sure that any supplement or medication is allowed. Even if a product claims to be "legal," contamination or hidden ingredients can lead to positive tests.

9. Supplements with Peptides

In supplement stores or online, you might see items labeled to "boost muscle growth" or "repair tissue fast," mentioning peptides. Some are protein powders that might include smaller peptides. Others could be claimed to be specialized performance enhancers. Buyers should be cautious:

1. **Quality Control**: Some products may have inaccurate ingredient lists.
2. **Hidden Banned Substances**: Even if the label does not say it contains banned peptides, contamination can happen.
3. **Lack of Proven Data**: Many performance claims are not backed by large studies.

Athletes who compete under strict doping rules often avoid less-trusted supplements to reduce the risk of failing a drug test by accident. Certified products tested by third parties might be safer, but the risk of contamination is still there.

---

10. Collagen Peptides for Joint and Tissue Support

Not all peptide uses revolve around doping. Collagen peptides, which are widely sold in health stores, are often aimed at joint health or tissue support. Some athletes take these supplements hoping to improve tendon or ligament strength. The idea is that providing extra amino acids might help the body repair tissues under heavy stress.

Studies on collagen peptides have shown some possible improvements in joint comfort or minor benefits in building cartilage. While results differ, these products are not typically banned in sports because they do not strongly shift hormone levels or oxygen delivery. Many are considered safe, though proof of their effectiveness is still debated. If an athlete chooses to try collagen peptides, they should combine it with an overall good diet and training plan, rather than relying on it alone.

---

11. Recovery from Injuries

Injuries can cut short an athletic season. Speeding up recovery is a major goal for sports medicine. Some clinics and researchers study growth-factor peptides or platelet-rich plasma (PRP) treatments. PRP involves taking a person's own blood, concentrating the platelets (which can release growth factors), and injecting it back into the injured site. Though not always called a "peptide therapy," these growth factors often include small proteins and peptides that help healing.

For torn ligaments or muscle tears, certain peptide injections might be tested to see if they can help form new tissue faster. However, research is still mixed, and these methods can be expensive or limited to advanced clinics. Athletes should be sure any treatment is approved under sports regulations and is provided by qualified medical professionals.

12. The Risk of Overreliance

Using peptides to push the body too far can backfire. If a substance lets an athlete train harder than their tissues can handle safely, they might end up with overuse injuries. Also, artificially boosting muscle growth can stress joints that are not ready for higher loads. There is also the potential for organ stress, especially if hormones are involved.

Some athletes have faced serious health problems after using banned substances that were not well-studied. This reminds us that the body is a complicated system. Changing one aspect, like muscle repair rate, can cause other parts to become unbalanced.

13. Legal Peptide Therapies

Not every peptide that athletes use is banned. Some may be permitted as normal medical treatments that do not directly increase performance. For example, a peptide might be used to help with gut health or to manage mild joint inflammation without significantly boosting speed or strength. While these legal peptides might not offer big performance gains, they can still assist overall wellness.

Athletes must keep an eye on any updates to anti-doping lists to ensure that their chosen therapy is still allowed. A substance can be permitted one year and restricted the next if evidence shows it offers a performance advantage beyond normal training or threatens health.

14. Natural Ways to Support Peptide Production

The body naturally makes many peptides that help in muscle building, recovery, and energy use. Athletes can enhance normal production by:

- **Eating Sufficient Protein**: Good sources include lean meats, fish, eggs, dairy, beans, and nuts.
- **Sleeping Enough**: Growth hormone and other repair signals often peak during deep sleep.
- **Doing Proper Workouts**: Strength training encourages muscle-building peptides. Endurance training promotes changes that help oxygen use.
- **Managing Stress**: Chronic stress can interfere with the normal hormone balance that includes peptide signals.

These methods are safe, usually accepted in all sports, and support the body's own ways of adapting to exercise. While they may not be as quick as injecting something, they lead to lasting improvements without the legal or health risks.

---

15. Youth Sports and the Danger of Early Peptide Use

In some regions, young athletes feel huge pressure to succeed. This can tempt them (or their coaches/parents) to try extreme shortcuts. Using hormones or peptides during the teenage years can disrupt normal growth patterns and cause harm. Sports associations strongly warn against giving young people any unapproved substances.

It is important for coaches and parents to foster a healthy approach to training. Good form, balanced diets, and a steady increase in workout intensity help the body develop in a safe way. If a teenager is genetically gifted in sports, their natural progress is often enough for them to reach high levels without risky substances.

---

16. Ethical Dimensions

Sports aim to measure natural talent combined with training and strategy. When an athlete takes a banned substance, they gain an advantage that many see as unfair. This is not just about personal health—it also affects the trust in sports events. If fans suspect doping, they might lose faith in the fairness of competitions.

Even legal peptides can raise questions if they give one athlete a large edge that is not available to others. As science advances, sports regulators must decide which methods cross the line into cheating. This debate is ongoing, and rules often try to keep up with new medical discoveries.

---

17. Examples of Commonly Discussed Peptides in Sports

1. **BPC-157**: Some claim it helps with healing and gut health. Research is limited, and it may be banned or unapproved.
2. **Thymosin Beta-4**: Linked to tissue repair. Also generally not allowed in organized sports.
3. **GHRP Family (Growth Hormone-Releasing Peptides)**: Encourage the body to release more growth hormone, thus banned in most competitions.
4. **IGF-1 LR3**: A modified form of IGF-1 that might enhance muscle growth, also usually banned.

There are many others sold online, often in forms with limited testing. Athletes risk doping violations if they try these unapproved substances.

---

18. Real-Life Stories of Peptide Use in Sports

Over the years, several high-profile doping cases have included peptides or growth factors. Some athletes faced suspensions or lost medals after tests or investigations proved they used banned peptides. These stories highlight that doping agencies watch for these substances, and breakthroughs in detection can happen even after an event has ended.

On the other hand, there are also accounts of medical uses for valid reasons. An athlete might get a permitted injection to help a serious tendon problem, with approval from officials. That can be part of legitimate treatment rather than cheating. The line between real medical need and performance gain can be blurry, which is why a strict process is in place for medical exemptions.

19. Practical Tips for Athletes Considering Peptides

1. **Check the Rules**: If you compete under an organization, look up the banned substance list or talk to a sports doctor.
2. **Consult Professionals**: A qualified sports physician or trainer can clarify the potential benefits, risks, and legality of any peptide.
3. **Be Skeptical of Claims**: If an online ad promises huge results with no downsides, be wary.
4. **Focus on Basics**: Solid training, rest, and nutrition often bring greater improvements over the long term than uncertain shortcuts.
5. **Keep Updated**: Rules and detection methods change. Something legal today might be banned tomorrow (or vice versa).

20. Summary: The Place of Peptides in Sports

Peptides can influence muscle recovery, endurance, and injury healing. These effects are why some athletes and trainers show interest in them. But many performance-enhancing peptides are banned due to fairness and health concerns. While there are legal uses for certain medical conditions, any attempt to use them for an unfair boost can lead to serious consequences.

Sports are built on competition within a shared set of rules. Athletes and supporters want to see talent, skill, and hard work on display. Peptides may have a role in recovery or joint health, but pushing into doping can harm both the athlete's body and the spirit of fair competition. In the end, balancing the potential benefits of peptide-based approaches with ethical and health concerns is a key task for sports communities around the world.

Moving forward, we will look at the rules and safety guidelines that surround peptides, so that anyone who might think of using them understands what is at stake and how to proceed responsibly.

Chapter 11: Regulations and Safety Guidelines

Peptides have gained more public attention as their uses expand across health, beauty, and wellness. With that interest comes a need for clear regulations and guidelines to ensure safety and protect consumers. In this chapter, we will go over how governing bodies watch over peptide products, the rules that guide their production and sale, and the steps that people can take to make better decisions when considering peptide use. We will also talk about why these rules matter, how they differ around the world, and what challenges remain in keeping peptides safe and effective for users.

---

1. Why Are Peptides Regulated?

Peptides are biologically active substances. This means they can cause changes in the body, for better or worse. Some are prescription drugs that require strict testing before they can be given to the public. Others are sold as supplements or found in cosmetics. Because peptides can have strong effects—on blood sugar, tissue repair, or even hormone balance—health authorities want to make sure that products containing peptides are made responsibly and do not harm consumers.

There is also the issue of false claims. Some products promise big results without real proof. People may spend money on something that does not work or, worse, may be unsafe. Regulations aim to keep low-quality or misleading products out of the market. They also help provide a process for checking side effects, correct labeling, and honesty about what a product can and cannot do.

---

2. Government Agencies Overseeing Peptides

In many countries, regulating peptide-based products involves multiple agencies or departments. For example, in the United States, the Food and Drug Administration (FDA) monitors drugs, medical devices, and certain types of supplements. In the European Union, agencies such as the European Medicines Agency (EMA) handle similar tasks, working with local groups in each member state.

When a peptide is used as a prescribed medicine—say, for balancing blood sugar in people who need that type of support—its maker must show proof of safety and effectiveness through data from scientific trials. The same holds true in other major markets such as Canada, Japan, and Australia, where local authorities like Health Canada or the Therapeutic Goods Administration (TGA) have rules requiring companies to run tests and share their results. This process can take many years and cost a lot of money.

On the other hand, if a peptide is included in a cosmetic product or sold as a supplement, the path to market can be different. Certain countries have less strict rules for supplements or cosmetics than for medicines. This difference means some peptide products reach consumers with fewer requirements for proof. Still, these products must typically follow rules on labeling, purity, and safety checks.

---

3. Pharmaceutical-Grade vs. Other Peptides

Peptides often come in different "grades" based on their intended use. Pharmaceutical-grade peptides are made to meet strict standards of purity and consistency. They are created in facilities that follow "Good Manufacturing Practices" (GMP), which means each step of production is carefully controlled and documented. This lessens the chance of contamination or mix-ups. If a peptide is meant to treat a health condition, it will usually be made under GMP conditions.

In contrast, research-grade peptides are sold for lab tests. These are generally not meant for human use and might not meet the highest purity standards. There are also peptide products marketed as "cosmetic-grade" or included as active ingredients in creams or lotions. Such products may or may not be made to GMP standards, depending on the company. The lack of universal definitions for "research-grade," "cosmetic-grade," or similar labels can cause confusion among buyers. That is why many experts suggest verifying that a product follows recognized quality standards if it is intended for human use.

---

4. Prescription vs. Over-the-Counter

If a peptide is classified as a prescription drug, doctors must approve it for patients who need it for a specific medical purpose. Examples include certain peptide-based treatments for diabetes or growth-related issues. In these cases, the drug has gone through clinical trials to show it meets standards of safety and effectiveness for that condition. A pharmacist then dispenses it, and the patient uses it under a doctor's supervision.

Meanwhile, some peptide items are sold over-the-counter (OTC) or online without a prescription. They might be labeled as dietary supplements or cosmetic products. While these can be legally sold in some places, they do not always have the same level of safety data behind them. Some might be perfectly fine, but others could be subpar or even contaminated. Because many of these OTC peptides do not require official approval before being sold (in regions where local laws allow this), consumers have to do more homework when picking which products to trust.

---

5. Labeling and Advertising Claims

Product labels and marketing should be honest about what is inside a product and what it can do. In many countries, companies that sell peptide-based products must follow rules that limit what they can claim. If they say their product treats or cures a disease, that usually places the product into the "drug" category, which then demands stringent testing.

For products classified as cosmetics or supplements, the rules tend to be looser. They are allowed to say things like "supports healthy skin" or "may help keep nails strong," but they cannot legally declare the product "cures" or "prevents" diseases without special approval. In reality, some labels still make big, unproven statements, which can mislead buyers. Agencies try to watch for these but do not always catch them all. Shoppers should be cautious with marketing claims that sound too good to be true.

6. Rules Vary by Region

Each country has its own laws about peptides. While there are similarities, there can be noticeable differences in how tightly these items are controlled. For instance, one nation might require a prescription for a certain peptide, while another might allow it to be sold freely if labeled as a supplement. The same product could be legal in one place and banned in another.

Some countries are still developing specific regulations. Because peptide science has grown quickly, lawmakers might not have detailed rules on every new product. They may rely on broader legislation for drugs, food, or cosmetics. In these cases, companies can sometimes exploit gray areas, leading to a flood of new peptides on the market. Buyers who shop internationally need to keep in mind that local regulations may not protect them if the product is imported from a place with weak oversight.

---

7. Safety Concerns with Unregulated Products

A big worry in the peptide market is the presence of unregulated or counterfeit items. When a product is not tested or inspected, several things can go wrong:

1. **Contamination**: Poor manufacturing conditions can let harmful substances or germs get into the final product.
2. **Wrong Dosage**: The product might have less or more of the peptide than the label says, leading to poor results or unexpected side effects.
3. **Harmful Additives**: Sometimes, unapproved fillers or chemicals are added to lower costs or alter how the product looks.
4. **Fake Products**: Unscrupulous sellers may claim to have a genuine peptide but are actually selling something else.

Any of these issues can cause health risks, from mild irritation to severe poisoning or long-term harm. That is why the first rule of peptide use is to choose sources that demonstrate care in how they produce and test their items.

8. Online Market and Black Market Worries

Peptide products are widely sold on the internet. Many sites promise advanced formulas or special peptides that claim amazing results. But the anonymity of online commerce lets dishonest businesses operate without being tracked easily. Some might ship products that do not match what was advertised, label them incorrectly, or skip quality checks altogether.

Black market sales of prescription peptides also occur, especially those sought for body enhancement or sports performance. These can come from overseas labs with questionable standards, or they might even be stolen from legitimate sources and resold. Using such black market products is very risky. It can lead to doping violations if the peptides are banned in sports, but also to severe health consequences if the product is tainted or formulated improperly. Authorities in many countries try to clamp down on these black market channels, but the online environment can be hard to police.

---

9. Doping Policies and Peptides

A specialized area of peptide regulation involves sports. Groups that set rules for athletes, such as the World Anti-Doping Agency (WADA), keep track of many banned peptides. They do this because some peptides can boost muscle building, improve endurance, or help with recovery in ways that offer an unfair advantage. Athletes caught using these banned substances can face suspensions or other penalties.

At the same time, there can be peptides that are not on banned lists and might be used for basic health or skin care. Sports authorities update their rules often, so athletes must be very cautious with any peptide-based product, even a cosmetic one, to ensure it does not contain banned chemicals. They often consult medical experts who know the latest doping rules.

---

10. Good Manufacturing Practices (GMP)

A cornerstone of safe peptide production is adherence to Good Manufacturing Practices. GMP standards demand that producers follow strict protocols to prevent contamination, ensure consistent dosing, and document every step. Factories must have clean rooms, trained staff, and procedures for testing raw materials. Each lot of a product should be traced, and if a problem is found, it can be recalled.

Companies that meet GMP standards usually share this information to build trust. Buyers can look for certifications on labels or on the company's website. While GMP does not guarantee a product works as advertised, it does show that basic production quality standards have been followed. This lowers the risk of faulty or unsafe products.

11. Testing, Recalls, and Post-Market Surveillance

For prescription peptides, the journey to market includes multiple levels of testing. First, there is lab work, then animal studies, and finally clinical trials with human participants. Once a peptide-based drug is approved, agencies might still keep an eye on it for rare side effects that appear in the broader population. If problems come up, regulators can require changes in labeling, add warnings, or even pull the drug from the market.

Cosmetic and supplement peptides often have a lighter approval process. Still, if a pattern of harmful side effects emerges, authorities can step in. In many countries, public health agencies run systems where doctors or consumers report issues tied to a product. These reports can lead to an investigation, product tests, or recalls if a serious threat is found. The big challenge, however, is that such systems depend on people noticing and reporting problems. If few people report, a harmful product might stay on the market longer than it should.

12. Ethical and Legal Responsibilities

Companies that sell peptide products have moral and legal obligations to offer safe, honest goods. This includes:

1. **Accurate Labeling**: Listing all active peptides and any other key ingredients.
2. **Truthful Advertising**: Not overstating benefits or hiding known risks.

3. **Compliance with Local Laws**: Following the guidelines wherever they sell the product.
4. **Continuous Monitoring**: Watching customer feedback and being ready to recall items if new safety concerns arise.

On the consumer side, there is a responsibility to use products as directed. If a peptide cream says "apply once a day," using it five times a day may lead to irritation or worse. If a supplement says it is not for pregnant women, ignoring that warning can be risky. Personal research and a cautious mindset help people avoid making choices that could harm them.

13. Seeking Professional Advice

Because peptides can affect biological processes, it is wise to consult health professionals when thinking of using them, especially if the peptides claim to alter hormones, growth, or other critical body functions. A doctor, pharmacist, or nurse with knowledge of peptides can give advice on safety, correct dosage, and possible interactions with medications. They may also suggest medical tests to check if a particular peptide is suitable. For instance, some peptides can affect blood sugar or thyroid function, so skipping a medical evaluation could lead to unexpected problems.

For cosmetic peptides, a dermatologist can help figure out if a certain product is likely to be helpful or if its claims are more marketing than science. Checking with a professional is especially important for people who have allergies, skin conditions, or other ongoing health issues.

14. Points to Check Before Buying a Peptide Product

1. **Reputation of Manufacturer**: Does the company have a track record of quality? Are they transparent about their production and testing?
2. **Certifications**: Look for GMP or third-party testing labels. These indicate higher standards of production.
3. **Ingredient List**: Make sure the peptide is clearly named. Watch for excessive fillers or unidentified chemicals.

4. **Claims and Promises**: If the seller claims the product "fixes everything" or shows "overnight miracles," be skeptical.
5. **Refund or Return Policies**: Reputable companies usually have reasonable policies if the product fails to meet expectations.

---

15. Safety Steps for Personal Use

After buying a peptide product, the following steps can help lower risk:

- **Start Low and Go Slow**: If it is a supplement or topical product, consider starting with a low dose or small skin test to check for reactions.
- **Watch for Side Effects**: Any unusual swelling, nausea, fatigue, or other symptoms could mean the product is not suitable.
- **Keep Records**: Note the dates and amounts used. This can help a doctor pinpoint the cause if problems develop later.
- **Store Properly**: Some peptides require refrigeration or protection from light. Follow the label or ask the company for storage instructions.
- **Avoid Mixing**: Combining multiple peptides or other strong supplements can be risky unless done under expert guidance.

---

16. The Role of Professional Organizations

Professional groups in fields like pharmacy, dermatology, and sports medicine often release guidelines or position statements on peptide use. They might highlight best practices, warn about emerging risks, or remind members of ethical responsibilities. For instance, a sports medicine board might alert doctors about new peptides used in doping, encouraging them to be watchful when treating athletes.

Some associations also educate the public through websites or brochures. They may explain the difference between regulated and unregulated products, how to spot suspect marketing, or when to seek a prescription. These efforts help people navigate a market that can be confusing.

17. Monitoring Global Trade

Because peptides are sold across borders, agencies sometimes work together to prevent illegal shipments. Customs officials may seize shipments of peptides that do not meet local requirements or appear counterfeit. International police organizations share data on suspicious exporters or distributors. Despite these efforts, the sheer volume of global e-commerce makes full enforcement challenging.

If a consumer orders peptides from another country, they might accidentally break import laws. In some cases, the product could be seized at customs. Even if it arrives, there is no guarantee that local regulations were followed in making that product. This highlights the complexity of the international peptide market.

---

18. Ongoing Challenges in Regulation

The rapid pace of scientific advances creates a continuous challenge. New peptides may appear faster than lawmakers can evaluate them. Smaller companies might rush to sell novel peptides, citing preliminary studies that have not been confirmed by larger research or clinical trials. Lawmakers must decide whether to ban or closely monitor new peptides right away, or allow some flexibility for innovation. Striking this balance can be hard.

Another issue is how to handle "off-label" use. A doctor might prescribe a certain peptide for a condition that is not officially approved but is supported by some clinical evidence. This practice can help patients who have no other options, but it can also be misused if done without proper oversight. Regulators try to keep track of patterns in off-label prescriptions to catch potential abuses or safety problems.

---

19. Moving Toward Better Standards

Many experts want clearer global standards for peptides, rather than a patchwork of national rules. Such standards could require at least a basic level of testing, labeling, and manufacturing quality. They might also create shared lists of banned or restricted peptides, making it easier to stop illegal trade. However, achieving global agreement on these points is no small feat due to economic and political differences between nations.

Meanwhile, education is a key tool. If more people know how to spot questionable products and understand why certain guidelines exist, they are less likely to buy unsafe items. Medical and pharmacy schools now include lessons on emerging therapies, including peptides, so that new professionals can guide the public responsibly.

20. Conclusion: Staying Safe and Informed

Regulations and guidelines exist to protect users of peptide products, though the rules can be complex and vary widely by region. From prescription drugs to everyday cosmetic creams, peptides come in many forms, and each form has a different regulatory path. By paying attention to labeling, certifications, and official sources of advice, consumers can lower their risks and get the most out of what peptides have to offer.

Safety guidelines, meanwhile, continue to evolve as new peptides appear in medicine, beauty, and other fields. Authorities want to keep up with scientific discoveries while preventing harm and stopping dishonest practices. In the end, well-structured regulations and informed consumers form the backbone of a safer, more trustworthy peptide market. People who wish to use these products should remain alert, ask questions, and rely on credible sources rather than gimmicks or gray-market deals. This careful approach helps ensure that peptides are used in a responsible way that respects both personal health and the broader public good.

Chapter 12: Research and Clinical Trials

Science never stops exploring the potential of peptides. In labs around the world, researchers look at how these small chains of amino acids can be harnessed for new medical treatments, improved beauty products, or better ways to support health. To turn a promising peptide into a real-world product, however, it must go through thorough investigation. Clinical trials are a key step in this process, providing evidence about a product's safety and results. In this chapter, we will outline how peptide research typically unfolds, from early lab studies to the trials that determine if a new therapy or solution reaches the public.

---

1. Early Discovery: Searching for New Peptides

Scientists find new peptides in various places: plants, animals, bacteria, or even in the human body. A key motivation is that peptides often have very specific actions. They can lock onto certain receptors or carry signals with greater precision than many older drugs. Sometimes, researchers isolate a peptide from a natural source—like a marine organism—to see if it has potential in fighting infections or encouraging tissue repair.

Modern technology helps this search. High-speed screening tools allow researchers to test thousands of molecules for interesting effects. Computers can also help predict how a new peptide might fold or bind to targets. By sorting through enormous data sets, scientists can zero in on peptides that look like good candidates for further study.

---

2. Designing Synthetic Peptides

Once a peptide with beneficial properties is discovered, researchers might create synthetic versions in the lab. These copies can be adjusted by changing a few amino acids or adding small modifications that make the peptide more stable. For instance, one might add a special chemical group that stops enzymes from breaking the peptide down too fast. Or they might replace certain amino acids with unusual versions that boost its ability to stay active in the bloodstream.

This design process is often guided by computer models, which show how a peptide might fold or interact with a target. Lab tests then confirm which modifications help and which do not. By going through several design cycles, researchers can create a refined version of the original peptide—one that is more potent, more stable, and less likely to cause issues.

3. Preclinical Testing: Lab and Animal Studies

After finalizing a promising peptide, scientists move into the preclinical stage. This involves:

1. **Cell Culture Tests**: The peptide is tested on cells grown in dishes to see if it does what it is meant to do. For example, if it is supposed to help wound healing, researchers might apply it to cultured skin cells and measure cell growth or protein production.
2. **Toxicity Screens**: Even if a peptide seems safe, it must be checked for harmful effects. This might include seeing if it harms normal cells or if it triggers abnormal reactions.
3. **Animal Studies**: Small animals like mice or rats may receive the peptide to see how it behaves in a living system. Researchers note if it reduces disease symptoms or causes side effects. They also look at how the peptide is absorbed, distributed, and excreted.

These steps provide early safety data and show if the peptide is on track for real benefits. If significant problems come up—like organ damage or severe immune responses—the project may be halted or revised. However, if results are encouraging, the team can request permission to test the peptide in humans.

4. The Role of Ethics Committees

Before clinical trials in humans can start, an independent ethics committee or review board must approve the plan. These groups exist to protect the rights and well-being of volunteers. They examine details of the proposed study: the number of participants, the dose of the peptide, possible risks, and how researchers will inform participants about these risks.

The ethics committee checks that the study does not place people in undue danger or breach their privacy. It also looks at the scientific basis—if the preclinical work is too shaky, or if the researchers cannot explain the point of the trial, it might be denied. This layer of oversight is critical for making sure that research meets moral and scientific standards.

5. Phase I Clinical Trials: First-in-Human Tests

Phase I is where people first receive the experimental peptide. Usually, these volunteers are healthy adults, though sometimes patients with a certain condition are included if the risks are too high for healthy volunteers. The main goal is to assess safety and see how the body handles the peptide. Researchers track side effects, measure how quickly the peptide is metabolized, and see if it stays at effective levels in the bloodstream.

Phase I trials are small, often involving fewer than 100 participants. Because everything is new at this stage, close monitoring is essential. If the peptide proves safe and well-tolerated in Phase I, the research can move on to the next phase.

6. Phase II Clinical Trials: Testing Efficacy and Dose

Phase II trials focus on whether the peptide actually helps the condition it is meant to target. They also refine the best dose. These studies can involve a few hundred patients who have the relevant medical issue. Researchers typically divide them into groups that get different doses or a placebo. By comparing results, they learn if the peptide improves symptoms, how well it compares to standard treatments (if any), and what side effects appear at different doses.

Phase II can last months or even years, depending on how quickly the condition changes. Scientists also watch for any problems that did not surface in Phase I. If the peptide shows a positive effect without serious harm, the work can move on to Phase III.

7. Phase III Clinical Trials: Large-Scale Confirmation

Phase III is the biggest, most complex step before a peptide drug can gain approval. It can involve hundreds or thousands of patients in multiple clinics or hospitals. The aim is to confirm that the peptide works better than a placebo or current standard treatment, and to gather more safety data across a diverse population.

At this stage, researchers also study how the peptide interacts with other drugs that people might already be taking. They analyze data to see if certain subgroups—like older adults or those with other illnesses—have a different response. Phase III trials are costly but crucial for proving that the peptide has real-world benefits that outweigh any risks. If successful, the results of Phase III often form the core of an application to health authorities seeking official approval to market the peptide.

---

8. Regulatory Submission and Approval

After Phase III, a company or research group compiles all data into a dossier and submits it to the relevant authorities (like the FDA in the U.S. or EMA in Europe). The dossier includes:

- **Clinical Trial Data**: Summaries of Phase I, II, and III results, showing how safe and effective the peptide is.
- **Manufacturing Details**: Explanation of the production process, purity standards, and stability data.
- **Labeling Plans**: Proposed instructions for doctors or patients, including dosage guidelines, warnings, and possible side effects.

Experts at the agency review this massive amount of information, sometimes convening advisory panels that include outside specialists. The review can take months or years. If the product meets all the requirements, it may get approved. Some peptides receive approval for limited use first, especially for serious conditions where few treatments exist. This is known as "conditional" or "accelerated" approval, meaning ongoing data collection must continue to confirm benefits.

9. Post-Approval Monitoring

Gaining approval does not mean research is over. Authorities often require post-marketing studies or Phase IV trials to look at the peptide's long-term effects in a larger population. This can reveal rare side effects that did not appear in earlier phases. For example, a risk that shows up in only 1 out of 10,000 people might be missed in smaller studies but become apparent when millions start using the peptide.

Companies may also test the peptide for other uses. For instance, a peptide first approved for one type of wound healing might show promise in another type of tissue repair. In such cases, they might run new trials and seek additional approvals. This ongoing process helps refine how and when the peptide is used, often improving safety labels or updating dosage recommendations.

---

10. Research on Cosmetic Peptides

Not all peptides end up as prescription drugs. Some are geared for cosmetics or over-the-counter products. The research approach may be different, often less strict than for medicines. However, serious companies still do basic safety and effectiveness tests. They might check how well a peptide cream penetrates the skin, or whether it helps with hydration or signs of aging.

Though not required to run the same level of trials as a new drug, some cosmetic peptide makers hire clinical testing labs to gather data. For example, they might run a double-blind test comparing a peptide cream to a dummy cream. Volunteers might use the product for several weeks while researchers measure skin firmness or dryness. This type of study can give real evidence about the product's value. Yet, because the bar for cosmetic approval is lower than for drugs, many products reach the market with minimal data.

---

11. Nutritional Peptides: Another Branch of Research

As interest in functional foods grows, some researchers look at peptides that come from everyday foods. These peptides might be formed when proteins are digested or fermented, and they could support health in subtle ways—such as aiding digestion or helping maintain normal blood pressure. Verifying these benefits needs a different research path, often involving dietary studies where participants consume foods or supplements containing the peptide. Over time, scientists measure changes in markers like blood pressure or cholesterol.

Such studies can be tricky because diet is complex. People eat many different things, and controlling all variables is difficult. But with good design, these trials can show whether a particular dietary peptide truly has a benefit beyond basic nutrition.

---

12. Challenges in Peptide Clinical Research

Despite their promise, peptide-based trials face unique hurdles:

- **Stability**: Many peptides break down quickly in the body, so researchers must find ways to protect them or deliver them effectively.
- **Cost**: Synthetic production or large-scale isolation can be expensive, raising the price of trials.
- **Patient Compliance**: If a peptide must be injected often, some volunteers might drop out of the study, making it harder to collect complete data.
- **Complexity of Action**: Peptides can act on multiple receptors or pathways, making it tricky to pinpoint side effects or interactions.

Researchers work around these challenges by designing better formulations, using advanced delivery methods (like slow-release injections or special coatings for pills), and carefully selecting volunteers who are most likely to show measurable results.

---

13. Breakthrough Areas

Several fields of medicine and health are especially active in peptide research:

1. **Metabolic Disorders**: Peptides that regulate blood sugar or appetite are an active area, with new variants of known hormones being tested for weight and glucose control.

2. **Infection Control**: Antimicrobial peptides that target drug-resistant bacteria hold promise. Some labs test these peptides to see if they can avoid the pitfalls of typical antibiotics.
3. **Cancer Therapy**: Peptides can be designed to hit cancer cells while sparing healthy ones, or to help the immune system spot tumors more effectively.
4. **Wound Healing**: Short amino-acid chains that promote tissue repair, reduce scarring, or speed up healing are under investigation for burns and chronic wounds.
5. **Neurological Issues**: Some peptides might support nerve cell function or protect brain cells, though crossing the blood-brain barrier remains a challenge.

In each of these fields, clinical trials are moving forward, hoping to offer new treatments where older ones fall short.

14. Funding and Collaboration

Developing a peptide from idea to approval can cost millions or even hundreds of millions of dollars. As a result, many labs partner with pharmaceutical firms or government agencies that supply grants. Universities play a major role, often spinning off start-up companies around promising discoveries. Some philanthropic organizations also back peptide research, especially for conditions with few treatment options.

Collaborations between academic teams, private companies, and public funding bodies can speed up research by letting each group contribute expertise. A university lab might focus on early-stage discovery, while an industry partner handles large-scale production and marketing. However, these partnerships must also handle questions of intellectual property and profit-sharing fairly.

15. The Rise of Personalized Peptides

Researchers are exploring the idea of creating peptides tailored to an individual's genetic or biological profile. This is part of "personalized medicine," which aims to deliver treatments that are more effective for a given patient. For instance, if a person's tumor has a specific receptor, a peptide might be built or selected to bind just that receptor. Early clinical trials are testing whether such custom approaches can improve outcomes.

Personalized peptides might also be used for rare diseases where the usual "one-size-fits-all" medication does not work well. By adjusting the amino-acid sequence, labs can build peptides that target unusual variations in a patient's cells. While still early-stage, this line of research hints at a future where each person might receive a unique therapy based on their biology.

---

16. Clinical Trial Transparency

In recent years, there has been a push for more openness in reporting clinical trial results. People want to see that negative or neutral results are shared, not just the positive ones. This helps avoid a skewed view of a peptide's potential. In many countries, rules now require registering a trial before it starts, posting its design, and later sharing findings. This transparency reduces the chance that companies will hide studies where a peptide did not work as hoped.

Public registries let scientists and others track how many peptide trials are ongoing, which conditions they address, and whether the results match the initial claims. This also helps prevent researchers from duplicating the same work unknowingly, saving time and money.

---

17. Real-World Examples of Successful Peptide Therapies

Over the last few decades, several peptide-based drugs have won approval. These real-world successes show how the research and trial process can pay off:

- **GLP-1 Agonists**: Widely prescribed for sugar balance, they went through rigorous Phase I-III studies before hitting the market. New versions keep appearing, each with improved delivery or fewer side effects.
- **Calcitonin**: Used for bone conditions in certain populations. It demonstrated benefits in controlled trials, leading to its acceptance as a treatment option.

- **Somatostatin Analogs**: Helpful for issues involving hormone secretion. Their path through clinical trials showcased how changing a natural peptide slightly can yield a stable, effective therapy.

These examples remind us that, while the development path is long and expensive, it can lead to valuable medical tools that help many people.

---

18. Shortcomings of Current Trials

Despite improvements, clinical trials do not solve every question:

- **Limited Diversity**: Sometimes, the volunteers in a trial might not represent the full population who will use the peptide. This can mask differences in how various groups respond.
- **Short Follow-Up**: Trials might track outcomes for a few months or years, but some side effects might only appear after longer use.
- **Cost Barriers**: High costs may discourage research on peptides that lack strong commercial promise, even if they could help smaller patient groups.
- **Complex Diseases**: Many disorders have multiple causes. A single peptide might help only part of the picture, needing combination approaches that are harder to test.

Researchers and regulators recognize these limits and look for ways to design better studies. For instance, adaptive trial designs can adjust the protocol as data emerges, speeding up or improving how new peptides are tested.

---

19. Future Directions

The future of peptide research and trials is shaped by:

- **Advanced Delivery Systems**: Nanoparticles or skin patches might allow peptides to be delivered without injections, boosting patient comfort.
- **Computational Biology**: More powerful software can predict peptide structure and function, cutting down on trial-and-error in the lab.

- **Gene Editing Links**: Some scientists experiment with using peptides alongside gene-editing tools to target illnesses at the genetic level.
- **Global Collaboration**: As knowledge grows, labs around the world may work together, sharing data more openly to speed discovery and reduce duplicate work.

All these trends point toward a landscape where peptides become even more central in medicine, but also in wellness and cosmetic fields.

---

20. Putting It All Together

From the lab bench to large-scale human trials, the process of bringing a peptide from idea to everyday use is thorough and cautious. It needs teamwork among researchers, doctors, volunteers, regulators, and more. The clinical trial phases ensure that a new peptide is not only effective but also safe enough for wide use. While some cosmetic or food-based peptides undergo less intensive testing, reputable brands still seek evidence to back their claims.

For the public, it is helpful to understand these steps. When a product says "clinically tested," people can ask: which clinical phase, and how big were the trials? If a supplement is described as "groundbreaking" but has no published data, that raises questions. With so many peptides being studied, some will advance and transform parts of health care, while others will fade away after failing to prove themselves in trials.

In the end, research on peptides is a field full of promise—across diseases, cosmetic improvements, and nutritional approaches. Clinical trials stand at the heart of that promise, separating truly beneficial discoveries from mere hype. As science keeps moving, those who watch developments in peptide research can look forward to new and improved products, guided by solid evidence rather than guesswork.

Chapter 13: Peptides and Mental Health

Peptides are small chains of amino acids that take part in many body functions, including those that involve the brain and mind. While people often focus on how peptides help with issues like wound healing or muscle growth, these tiny molecules can also guide signals that shape our thoughts, feelings, and behavior. In this chapter, we will look at how peptides connect to mental health, why some of them influence moods or stress, and what experts are learning about possible treatments. We will also talk about what is still unknown and what challenges exist in using peptides to help manage conditions like depression, anxiety, or other mental problems.

1. The Brain as a Network of Signals

The brain is a complex network where billions of cells communicate through electrical and chemical signals. Among these chemical signals, some are small molecules known as neurotransmitters (like serotonin or dopamine), while others are slightly bigger molecules called neuropeptides. Neuropeptides are peptides that specifically act in the brain or nervous system. They can send or shape signals between neurons, influencing how we sense the world and how we respond to it.

In many cases, a neuropeptide is released by one neuron and moves across a tiny gap to another neuron. The second neuron has receptors that match the shape of the peptide, and once the peptide binds, it sets off certain processes. These processes might make the neuron more or less likely to send its own signals. This is one way the brain fine-tunes mood, memory, and stress responses.

Neuropeptides often work alongside the classic neurotransmitters. They can adjust how strongly a signal is felt, or how long it lasts. Because they often have more complex shapes and can interact with specialized receptors, they can create very focused effects in specific regions of the brain. This can lead to subtle changes in mood or behavior that are different from those caused by more common messengers like serotonin alone.

2. Types of Brain-Related Peptides

Scientists have found many neuropeptides that play roles in mental health. A few examples include:

1. **Substance P**: Known mostly for sending pain signals, it also plays a part in mood and stress. If too much substance P is around, it might raise anxiety or stress responses.
2. **Neuropeptide Y (NPY)**: Linked to appetite and stress management. High levels of NPY can help calm stress signals, while low levels might lead to more anxious responses.
3. **Oxytocin**: Sometimes called the "bonding hormone." It is a peptide that, when released in the brain, might boost feelings of social connection or trust.
4. **Vasopressin**: Another peptide hormone involved in fluid balance, but in the brain, it can play a part in social behavior and stress.
5. **Corticotropin-Releasing Hormone (CRH)**: A peptide that starts the release of stress hormones in the body. If CRH levels are too high, it can lead to an overactive stress response.
6. **Beta-Endorphin**: A peptide that can reduce pain and stress, often linked to "feel-good" feelings in certain situations.

While each of these has specific roles, they overlap a lot. For example, peptides that manage stress also might shape mood or influence how the brain responds to pleasurable experiences.

---

3. Peptides in Mood Disorders

Mood disorders include depression, bipolar disorder, and related conditions. They may develop when certain signals in the brain are too strong, too weak, or out of balance. Traditional approaches often focus on neurotransmitters like serotonin or norepinephrine. However, some researchers think that neuropeptides could also be key players in the ups and downs of mood.

For example, substance P has attracted interest because blocking its activity in certain brain pathways may reduce signs of depression or anxiety in animal studies. Though trials in humans have had mixed outcomes, the link suggests that adjusting peptide levels could one day help. Other peptides like NPY might also guard against the negative effects of stress, which is often tied to depression.

Researchers are still exploring these ideas, but the potential is clear: if we can fine-tune neuropeptide systems, we might offer new options for those who do not respond well to usual antidepressants. That said, it is a tricky task, because these peptides can have multiple roles in different parts of the body. Blocking or boosting a peptide might help one function but cause problems somewhere else.

---

4. Peptides and Anxiety-Related Conditions

Anxiety can appear as nervousness, worry, or fear that is out of proportion to actual risks. The body's "fight or flight" response can become overactive, leading to both mental distress and physical changes like a faster heartbeat. Peptides often play important roles in turning these responses on or off.

Some studies highlight the role of corticotropin-releasing hormone (CRH) in anxiety. CRH triggers the release of cortisol, a major stress hormone. In normal amounts, cortisol helps us handle challenges, but if CRH is always high, it can keep the body in a constant state of alert, raising anxiety or panic. Researchers have looked at CRH-blocking drugs to see if they help ease anxiety or post-traumatic stress. Results are still preliminary, and more data is needed, but it points to a strong link between peptides and anxious thinking.

Neuropeptide Y is the opposite in some ways. It seems to calm stress reactions. In animals, higher levels of NPY in certain brain areas can lower anxious behavior. If scientists figure out how to boost NPY properly in people, it might offer a method to manage anxiety or stress that does not respond well to other treatments.

---

5. The Role of Stress and the Stress Axis

Stress is a normal reaction that can help people handle short-term challenges, but chronic stress can harm mental health. The hypothalamic-pituitary-adrenal (HPA) axis is central to the stress response, and many of its signals are peptides or peptide-related hormones. For instance, when the brain spots a threat, it releases CRH. CRH then triggers the pituitary gland to release another signal, which in turn prompts the adrenal glands to make cortisol. Cortisol helps the body get ready for action, but too much for too long can have negative effects.

If the HPA axis does not calm down, the brain might stay on high alert, fueling anxiety, depression, and even memory problems. Some experts propose that carefully guiding peptide signals in this axis could make the stress response more balanced. For instance, if there was a safe way to reduce CRH levels during chronic stress, it might help the body return to a calmer state. Research in this area is still early, though, and these peptides are involved in many bodily processes, so any therapy must avoid side effects.

---

6. Peptides for Social Behavior and Connection

Humans are social creatures, and certain neuropeptides shape how we bond with others. Oxytocin, for example, has long been studied for its effects on trust, empathy, and social bonding. Some small experiments in people suggest that oxytocin, given as a nasal spray, might help increase feelings of closeness or reduce social anxiety. However, these results can vary widely, and not everyone responds the same way.

Vasopressin, similar in structure to oxytocin, also appears to shape social behavior. Studies in animals show that changes in vasopressin can affect bonding patterns or aggression levels. Translating these findings into therapies for mental conditions—like certain types of social anxiety or conditions that involve trouble understanding social cues—remains a challenge. Still, it gives a clue as to how peptides might be used in the future to support social aspects of mental health.

---

7. Pain, Stress, and Emotions: The Substance P Example

Substance P is famous for carrying pain signals, but that is not all it does. In the brain, it might also influence fear or anxiety, especially in response to threats. If someone has very high levels of substance P in certain brain areas, it could amplify the emotional aspects of pain or worry. Blocking substance P in lab tests sometimes leads to a drop in anxious or stressed behaviors. Because of this, substance P has been explored as a possible target for new mood or anxiety treatments.

However, clinical trials in humans have shown mixed or limited success. Part of the reason may be that the brain's networks are extremely interlinked, and adjusting one signal can have ripple effects. It is also possible that only certain subgroups of patients would benefit, such as those with a specific type of anxiety or depression tied to overactive substance P signals. Researchers are still sorting out these details.

8. Post-Traumatic Stress and Peptide Pathways

Post-traumatic stress issues can arise after someone experiences or witnesses a severe or life-threatening event. Symptoms can include flashbacks, nightmares, and intense anxiety that does not go away easily. The brain's response to trauma involves many chemical messengers, including peptides. For example, CRH and substance P may increase after a traumatic event, making the person overly alert or ready for danger. Over time, this could lead to chronic fear or nightmares.

Some animal studies have tried blocking CRH or substance P to see if it reduces PTSD-like behavior. Results are encouraging in that they show a possible link. But turning this into a real treatment for humans is challenging, partly because every person's stress response and trauma experience is unique. A therapy that helps one group might not be as effective for another, or it might cause side effects that outweigh benefits.

9. Appetite, Eating Disorders, and Peptides

Peptides like NPY, ghrelin, and leptin are closely tied to appetite and body weight. But appetite and mood can link together, too. Emotional distress might lead some people to eat too much or too little, causing or worsening conditions like binge eating or anorexia. In some cases, these behaviors overlap with mood disorders such as depression or anxiety.

Researchers wonder if managing the body's hunger peptides could also help with emotional aspects of eating. For instance, high levels of ghrelin can drive hunger, but ghrelin also can affect mood. People with anorexia sometimes have higher ghrelin but do not feel hunger in the typical way, pointing to a broken link between the peptide and the emotional aspects of eating. While there is no simple fix, it shows that mental health, peptides, and appetite form a triangle that scientists are eager to better understand.

---

10. Delivery to the Brain: A Key Obstacle

One reason we do not see many peptide-based mental health treatments on the market is that delivering peptides to the brain is difficult. The blood-brain barrier is a strong border that protects the brain from harmful substances but also blocks many useful molecules, including most peptides. To help a peptide reach the brain, scientists must find special strategies like:

1. **Nasal Sprays**: The nasal route can let some molecules bypass parts of the blood-brain barrier. Oxytocin has been tested this way.
2. **Chemical Modifications**: Adding certain groups or changing amino acids to make the peptide more fat-soluble or less likely to be broken down.
3. **Nanoparticle Carriers**: Tiny carriers can slip through the blood-brain barrier, carrying the peptide inside until it reaches the brain.

Even with these methods, many peptides break down too quickly or fail to reach the areas where they are needed. This remains one of the largest obstacles to turning peptide research into real-world mental health therapies.

---

11. Current Treatments vs. Peptide Approaches

Common mental health treatments include talk therapy, lifestyle changes, and medications like selective serotonin reuptake inhibitors (SSRIs) or benzodiazepines. These can be effective but do not work for everyone. Peptides could provide new ways to target systems that these older drugs do not address. They might help if someone's condition involves stress signals or social bonding issues that are not improved by conventional medications.

Still, any new peptide-based treatment must go through the usual research process, including clinical trials. Because the brain is involved, safety is a major concern. A therapy that changes stress signals could help with anxiety, but if it also affects blood pressure or hormone release too much, it may not be viable. Trials also need to track subtle changes in mood or social behavior, which can be harder to measure than, say, a change in blood sugar.

12. Laboratory Findings and Human Trials

Much of what we know about peptides and mental health comes from animal studies, where researchers can precisely control conditions. Mice or rats may be bred to show anxiety-like behaviors, and then tested with peptide injections. Such studies reveal possible paths for new treatments. However, humans are more complex. A method that works in mice may not translate the same way for people.

A small number of human trials have tried things like CRH blockers, or NPY boosters, or oxytocin sprays. Some participants reported better stress handling or improved mood, but others showed little change. Results often differ by dosage, how the peptide is delivered, and whether the person has a specific type of mental health challenge. These differences make it tough to form universal conclusions. Nonetheless, each trial offers clues about how to refine the approach.

13. Personalized Medicine Hopes

Experts in mental health research often discuss "precision" or "personalized" medicine. This means tailoring therapies to each person's biology. Since peptides can target certain receptors, they might fit well into this personalized idea. For instance, if a person has very high CRH activity, a CRH-blocking peptide might help. If another person lacks enough NPY, then a therapy boosting NPY might be better.

Genetic tests or specific brain scans might one day let doctors see which peptide pathways are off balance in a patient. Then they could pick the matching peptide-based treatment. This approach would avoid the "trial and error" that often happens today, where patients might try one antidepressant or anti-anxiety drug after another, unsure of which will help. Of course, this personalized approach is still mostly in the future, given the complexity of mental health conditions.

14. Ethical and Social Questions

When we talk about using peptides to adjust mood, stress, or social interaction, ethical concerns appear. Would it be right to use a nasal spray that boosts trust or empathy in situations like sales negotiations or political debates? Could it be misused by those who want to manipulate people? Also, how do we make sure these therapies are used only for real mental health needs, not for gaining an unfair edge in certain settings?

Regulations around mental health drugs aim to ensure they are prescribed for genuine reasons. But peptides that affect social bonding might be simple to get if they are sold as "wellness" or "lifestyle" items. Society might need to discuss how best to handle these new tools before they become widely available.

15. Alternative Views: Behavioral Approaches

Some mental health experts warn against relying too heavily on drugs, whether they are peptides or classic medications. They argue that conditions like anxiety or depression often have psychological, social, or environmental causes that need talk therapy, social support, or changes in daily life. While peptides might help balance the chemical side, ignoring personal relationships, stress at work, or unresolved trauma might limit how much improvement someone can get.

A balanced perspective sees peptides, if proven safe and helpful, as one more option to combine with other strategies. It could be that in the future, a doctor might recommend short-term peptide therapy alongside counseling or lifestyle changes to help a person through a tough period. This integrated approach may lead to better outcomes than simply prescribing a medicine alone.

16. Over-the-Counter Supplements and Safety

Because peptides are popular, some products are sold online claiming to help mood or stress. They might include general peptides "for relaxation" or "for better focus." However, these items often lack solid clinical proof. Some may be mislabeled or mixed with unknown substances. People who buy them might not know the correct dosage or the potential side effects. Such unregulated use can lead to disappointment or harm.

If someone is interested in a peptide supplement for mental well-being, experts advise caution. Talking with a healthcare provider or mental health professional is smart, especially if the person already takes medication. Even if the supplement is labeled "natural," it can cause problems if it interacts with the body's systems or with other drugs in unexpected ways.

---

17. Possible Side Effects and Risks

When peptides target the brain, side effects could be wide-ranging, such as:

- **Too much sedation**: If a peptide overly calms certain signals, it could cause drowsiness or impaired thinking.
- **Hormonal imbalance**: Some peptides might also affect glands or hormones outside the brain, leading to weight changes, blood pressure issues, or sleep problems.
- **Emotional flattening**: If stress or excitement signals are reduced too much, a person might feel less engaged or enthusiastic.
- **Allergic reactions**: As with any peptide, there is a chance of allergic responses, though it is not very common.

Because the brain's networks are so complicated, it is not easy to predict how any one peptide will act in every individual. Clinical trials can flag the most common problems, but rare issues might appear only after widespread use. This is why regulation and close follow-up are critical.

18. Ongoing Studies and the Future

Many labs continue exploring peptides for mental health. Some focus on how to deliver them more reliably across the blood-brain barrier. Others look for brand-new peptides in nature that might calm stress or help with memory. A few projects aim to decode the exact role of certain neuropeptides in mental conditions, such as obsessive-compulsive disorder or borderline personality. While it is hard to predict which leads will become successful treatments, the range of research is large.

Experts say that in the coming years, we might see:

1. **Refined Oxytocin Sprays**: Possibly for autism-related social issues or certain anxiety situations.
2. **CRH Blockers**: For chronic stress or depression linked to high cortisol.
3. **NPY Enhancers**: To help with stress resilience, especially in people with trauma backgrounds.
4. **Targeted Injections**: Possibly delivered into certain brain regions for severe cases.

However, each of these ideas must still pass the test of scientific proof. It could take many more trials and some missteps before final forms of peptide-based mental health aids are widely used.

---

19. Tips for Curious Individuals

If you or someone you know is intrigued by peptides for mental well-being, keep these points in mind:

- **Seek Professional Guidance**: Talk to a mental health specialist or doctor, especially if you have a diagnosed condition or already use medications.
- **Watch for Evidence**: Look for products or therapies backed by clinical data. Ask for references to published studies, not just personal stories.
- **Be Realistic**: Understand that peptides are not magic cures. They may help in certain cases, but broad lifestyle factors and therapy can still play a big role in outcomes.

- **Stay Safe**: Avoid risky online products that do not disclose contents or proper dosing. If you choose to try any supplement, start with a small amount and watch for negative reactions.
- **Monitor Changes**: Keep track of any shifts in mood, sleep, or stress levels. Share updates with a healthcare professional to spot any side effects early.

20. Final Thoughts on Peptides and Mental Health

Peptides can serve as fine-tuned messengers in the brain, shaping feelings of stress, sadness, or social connection. They may offer new ways to help when usual treatments do not fully work. However, the science is still evolving. Though early findings show promise—like the potential of CRH blockers for stress or oxytocin for social anxiety—actual products are limited, and many remain in research or testing.

In the broader picture of mental health, peptides might one day fill gaps in our current options, giving doctors more targeted approaches to things like chronic stress, trauma, or social difficulties. Still, caution is essential. The brain's systems are deeply intricate, so even the best ideas can take years to become reliable and safe. For now, the best step for anyone dealing with mental health issues is to consult medical professionals, stay informed about new findings, and approach any untested product with care. Peptides could become part of a balanced approach to emotional well-being, but they are not a complete answer on their own.

Chapter 14: Peptide Manufacturing and Industry Practices

Peptides have many uses: they appear in prescription medications, skin care products, dietary supplements, and even in research labs. The process that leads from raw materials to a finished peptide-based product can be intricate. It involves high-level chemistry, rigorous testing, and attention to detail. In this chapter, we will look at how peptides are typically made, how companies handle quality control, and why industry standards like Good Manufacturing Practices (GMP) matter. We will also address some of the common pitfalls in the peptide industry, such as counterfeiting or impurities, and explore the future trends that might shape how peptides are produced on a large scale.

---

1. Reasons Behind Peptide Production

Scientists and manufacturers create peptides for many purposes. Pharmaceutical companies develop peptide-based drugs to treat conditions like diabetes, hormonal imbalances, or other problems. Cosmetic brands add peptides to serums and creams that claim to help with skin firmness or repair. Academic labs use peptides to study diseases or as tools to uncover how cells interact. Some health brands sell collagen peptide powders or other supplements for hair, skin, and nails. As a result, the global market for peptides has grown, spurring improvements in how they are made and inspected.

---

2. Basics of Peptide Synthesis

Peptides are chains of amino acids linked by peptide bonds. In living systems, the body uses ribosomes and RNA instructions to piece together these chains. In an industrial or laboratory setting, the process is typically reversed: scientists pick the order of amino acids they want, then join them step by step in a chemical reaction. This is usually done in two main ways:

1. **Solid-Phase Peptide Synthesis (SPPS)**
   This is the most popular method. The chain of amino acids grows while attached to a solid resin bead. The process goes in cycles:
   - An amino acid with a protective group is added.
   - A chemical reaction removes the protective group, letting the amino acid link to the chain.
   - Washes remove unreacted material.
   - The next amino acid is introduced.
     When the desired chain length is reached, the finished peptide is cut from the resin bead and further purified.
2. **Liquid-Phase Peptide Synthesis**
   Less common in modern large-scale factories but still used for certain specialized peptides. The idea is the same—link amino acids in the right order—but the steps happen in solution rather than on a solid support. It can be useful for smaller batches or for tricky sequences that do not work well on a resin.

Solid-phase synthesis speeds up the joining process since each new amino acid can be added in a controlled cycle. Machines can automate these steps, producing short peptides quickly. However, if the chain is very long, it can become more challenging, and yields might drop.

---

3. Protecting Groups and Purification

To ensure that each amino acid attaches in the correct spot, chemists use "protecting groups." These are small chemical shields placed on certain parts of the amino acid so it does not react at the wrong time. After each addition, they remove the protecting group from the newly added amino acid so the next link can form. This is a repetitive cycle, leading to a carefully assembled chain.

Once the full peptide is made, there is an additional purification step, often using techniques like high-performance liquid chromatography (HPLC). This step helps remove fragments that did not form correctly, leftover reagents, or other contaminants. The purity of a peptide can be stated as a percentage, like 95% or 99%. Medical or research-grade peptides often require very high purity, while cosmetic or nutritional peptides might be less strict, depending on their intended use.

4. Manufacturing Challenges

Peptide synthesis can run into several problems:

1. **Yield Declines**: If each amino acid addition is not close to 100% efficient, losses build up over a long chain. With 10 or 20 or more amino acids, the final yield might be lower than desired.
2. **Side Reactions**: Amino acids have chemical groups that might react in unintended ways, forming impurities.
3. **Complex Structures**: Some peptides have loops or special bonds (like disulfide bridges) that need extra steps to form correctly.
4. **Scalability**: Making a small sample in a lab is easier than producing large amounts consistently for commercial sale.

Overcoming these requires refining the chemical methods, carefully choosing solvents and reagents, and implementing strict monitoring. Companies that excel in peptide manufacturing invest in research to reduce costs, improve yields, and shorten production times.

---

5. Good Manufacturing Practices (GMP)

When peptides are made for use in medicines or certain regulated products, GMP standards often apply. GMP rules cover every detail, from how workers are trained to how the building is cleaned. They require:

- **Documented Processes**: Each batch must follow a written procedure, ensuring consistency.
- **Traceability**: Every ingredient, piece of equipment, and step is tracked. If a problem arises, the source can be found quickly.
- **Equipment Calibration**: Instruments like scales, chromatographs, or reactors must be regularly checked for accuracy.
- **Quality Checks**: Samples from each batch are tested to make sure they meet purity and identity standards. If a batch fails, it is discarded or reprocessed.

Following GMP can be expensive, but it helps guarantee that users get a product that is consistent and safe. This is crucial for prescription drugs, where a single error in dosage can risk lives. Even for cosmetic peptides, some companies opt for GMP-like procedures to assure customers about quality.

---

6. Quality Control and Testing

Proper quality control (QC) is vital throughout peptide manufacturing. Common tests include:

1. **Mass Spectrometry**: Checks the mass of the peptide to confirm it has the correct length and composition.
2. **HPLC Purity**: Measures how much of the product is the target peptide vs. impurities.
3. **Amino Acid Analysis**: Verifies the ratio of amino acids in the final product.
4. **Microbial Tests**: Ensures bacteria or other germs are not present, especially if the product is for injection or ingestion.
5. **Endotoxin Levels**: For injectable peptides, endotoxins (parts of bacteria) must be very low to prevent fevers or harmful reactions.

Each batch that passes these tests can be labeled with a certificate of analysis. This document details the results and any relevant specifications, helping buyers trust the product's authenticity.

---

7. The Rise of Large-Scale Manufacturing

As demand grows, more companies can produce large amounts of peptides. This is especially true for products like peptide-based drugs for blood sugar control or for some forms of hormonal support. Large biopharmaceutical plants might have specialized rooms where automated systems handle cycles of SPPS. After each run, they may produce several kilograms of a peptide with high purity.

Scaling up involves big investments in equipment and staff with specialized knowledge. It also requires tight supply-chain control of raw materials. Amino acids need to have minimal impurities to avoid spoiling the final product. Solvents must be high grade, and everything must be stored properly. Even small errors can waste a lot of material, costing thousands or even millions of dollars.

8. Differences Between Pharmaceutical and Cosmetic Grade

- **Pharmaceutical Grade**: Produced under strict conditions, with GMP oversight, extensive testing, and documentation. Must meet or exceed the purity, safety, and efficacy guidelines set by regulators.
- **Cosmetic Grade**: May not require the same level of regulation. The peptides might be pure enough for topical use but do not always reach the 99% or higher purity demanded by injectable or ingestible products. Labeling laws are often less strict, though reputable cosmetic brands still do stability and safety tests.

Because the cost of meeting pharmaceutical-grade standards is high, it is not practical for every type of peptide product. However, serious producers of cosmetic peptides often apply at least some GMP principles to gain consumer trust. In marketing, you might see claims like "produced in a GMP-certified facility," which indicates they follow certain guidelines even if the final product is not a prescription drug.

9. Counterfeit and Low-Quality Products

One problem in the peptide market is the presence of counterfeit or low-quality products. Some of these appear as "research peptides" sold online, claiming to match prescription-only items. They might use fancy names or claim lab testing, but in reality, they could be produced with cheap methods and contain unknown substances or incorrect sequences.

There have been cases where labs tested such items and found no real peptide or found harmful byproducts. These fake products can be especially dangerous if used by people who think they are buying something that mimics a legitimate drug. Besides health risks, it also hurts the reputation of honest peptide makers.

Buyers who want peptides for personal or research use should stick to well-known suppliers that share detailed testing data and have a good record. If a product's price seems too good to be true or if the seller will not provide a certificate of analysis, that is a red flag.

10. Sustainable and Green Approaches

Classic peptide synthesis often uses large volumes of chemicals, generating waste that must be disposed of safely. A push for "green chemistry" has led to attempts to reduce the environmental impact. Some labs explore methods that use less solvent, recycle materials, or rely on newer reactions that do not produce as many byproducts. They might also switch to more environmentally friendly protecting groups or reagents that degrade into harmless substances.

While these methods can help the planet, they also have to be efficient and cost-effective. The industry is gradually adopting more sustainable steps, though the change can be slow. Demand from clients for "eco-friendly" peptides could speed up this trend, as companies see it as a marketing advantage to highlight cleaner production processes.

11. Advanced Delivery Systems and Formulations

Making a pure peptide is only part of the puzzle—many peptides must also be formulated into a final product. This might be a pill, a cream, an injection, or a slow-release implant. Because peptides can break down easily, formulation scientists look for ways to protect them until they reach their target. Some approaches include:

- **Encapsulation**: Wrapping the peptide in microscopic carriers (like liposomes) to shield it from stomach acid or enzymes.
- **Depot Injections**: Designing an injection that releases the peptide slowly over days or weeks, reducing how often a patient needs a dose.
- **Transdermal Patches**: Placing the peptide in a patch that can pass it through the skin at a controlled rate.
- **Nasal Sprays**: Bypassing the gut so the peptide can enter the bloodstream or even approach the brain more easily.

These delivery strategies often call for advanced manufacturing steps, plus thorough stability and release-rate testing. The final product must maintain its potency and remain free of contaminants for as long as it is stored or used.

12. Automation and Robotics

Many big peptide factories use robots to carry out repetitive tasks. Automated synthesizers can measure out amino acids, deliver reagents, run wash cycles, and track the steps. This helps avoid human error and speeds up production. Automated systems can also handle tasks like weighing out raw materials, packaging, or applying labels.

Beyond saving time, automation keeps conditions consistent. Each batch can follow the same steps with minimal deviation. This leads to more uniform quality and lowers the chance of mistakes. Of course, skilled technicians and chemists remain essential to design recipes, fix issues, and interpret data.

---

13. Peptide Customization and Small Orders

While some factories focus on large batches of a few well-known peptides, others specialize in custom synthesis. A research lab or biotech start-up might need a unique sequence or a modified peptide for their experiments. These "on-demand" services can handle small orders of a few milligrams to grams, letting scientists explore new ideas without making huge quantities.

Custom orders often come with a higher price per gram, because setting up each batch takes time. The facility may also have to source special amino acid derivatives or add extra modifications (like fluorescent tags) that are not used in regular peptides. Still, custom synthesis is vital for innovation and for new products in development.

---

14. Intellectual Property and Licensing

Peptide sequences can be patented if they show novelty and provide a specific benefit. This means a company might have the exclusive right to produce or sell a certain peptide therapy for a set time. Others may pay licensing fees to use that peptide or combine it with other ingredients. Patent battles can arise if multiple groups claim ownership of similar sequences.

Sometimes, broad claims are made on a whole family of peptides, slowing research by requiring others to negotiate licenses. On the other hand, patent protection can encourage investors to fund the expensive work of bringing a new peptide to market. Balancing open science with legal rights remains a key discussion in the peptide field.

15. Global Peptide Manufacturing Hubs

Peptide production centers are found all around the world, but certain regions stand out. Countries like the United States, Germany, Switzerland, and China have large facilities that provide peptides for pharmaceutical and biotech clients. India has also emerged with manufacturers offering competitive prices. Each region has its own regulations, labor costs, and tax rules, so companies may choose to locate in the place that best suits their market focus.

With global transport links, peptides can be shipped anywhere, but time and temperature control matter. Many peptides need cold storage, so shipping can involve refrigerated containers or special packaging. This supply chain must be managed carefully to keep products from spoiling in transit.

16. Testing Beyond Purity: Activity and Stability

Even if a peptide is pure, it needs to show the intended activity. That means the chain must fold properly or bind to the right receptor. Some manufacturers provide extra data, like results from assays where the peptide is tested on cells that have the target receptor. This can confirm that the peptide is not just the right sequence but is also functional.

Stability is another factor. If a product sits in a warehouse for months, will it degrade? This is tested by storing samples at different temperatures and measuring changes in purity or activity over time. Based on the results, companies set expiration dates or specify storage needs, like "keep frozen at -20°C" or "stable at 4°C for six months."

17. Regulatory Oversight and Inspections

When peptides are sold as drugs, regulatory agencies like the FDA or EMA can inspect the factory. They check if the company follows GMP, keeps records properly, and tests the product thoroughly. If the factory does not meet standards, it can be cited for violations, forced to fix problems, or even shut down.

For peptides in cosmetics or supplements, oversight might be less strict, but there are still rules about safety and labeling. Some regions require registration or proof that products do not contain harmful levels of contaminants. Reputable makers often invite these inspections to show they operate responsibly.

---

18. Common Misunderstandings About Peptide Quality

- **High Purity Always Means Safe**: Even a 99% pure peptide can have harmful contaminants if that last 1% is toxic. Testing must look for specific dangerous impurities, not just measure overall purity.
- **All "Pharmaceutical Grade" Products Are Equal**: Some sellers misuse the term. Actual pharmaceutical-grade peptides have documentation and meet recognized standards.
- **If It Comes from a Lab, It Is Good**: Small labs might not follow GMP, and even well-intentioned scientists can slip up on QC. A recognized track record matters.

Consumers who want the best quality should look for clear evidence of manufacturing standards and test results, not just claims or brand names.

---

19. Future Directions in Peptide Manufacturing

Research in this field is moving at a fast pace. Potential trends include:

1. **Flow Chemistry**: Instead of doing the steps in separate batches, new machines might run a continuous flow where each amino acid addition happens in one pass, speeding up production.

2. **Green Solvents**: Shifting to less toxic or reusable solvents to reduce environmental harm.
3. **Enzyme-Assisted Synthesis**: Using enzymes can be gentler and more selective than harsh chemicals, possibly reducing side reactions.
4. **3D Printing of Peptides**: Early ideas suggest that specialized printers could build peptide arrays for research or screening, though it is still in the conceptual stage.
5. **AI and Machine Learning**: Helping scientists predict the best synthetic route or optimal conditions, trimming trial and error in making large or complicated peptides.

These advances could lower costs, improve yields, and bring new sequences to market faster. It could also open up the field to smaller players who want to innovate in niche areas.

---

20. Conclusion: Building Trust Through Quality

The success of the peptide industry rests on producing effective, safe, and consistent products. Whether it is a lifesaving drug, a lab reagent, or a cosmetic serum, buyers deserve confidence that the peptide meets its claims. This requires careful planning, precise chemistry, and strict oversight at every step. Good Manufacturing Practices and robust quality control help set a high bar that reputable firms strive to meet.

For consumers, knowing about these production methods and standards can help in choosing trustworthy brands. As science uncovers more uses for peptides—and as people become more interested in them—transparent, well-regulated manufacturing will stay important. In the best cases, it helps ensure that the promise of peptides is not overshadowed by concerns about contamination or false claims. By holding onto solid practices and embracing new technology, the peptide industry can continue to grow and serve many needs, from advanced medicine to everyday self-care.

Chapter 15: Misconceptions About Peptides

Peptides are short chains of amino acids that have many roles in the body. They appear in health news and product ads, often described in ways that may or may not be accurate. Because they are linked to subjects like beauty, weight, and muscle, it is easy for myths or half-truths to spread. In this chapter, we will look at some common misunderstandings about peptides. We will explain why each misconception exists and what the facts really are. Knowing these points can help people avoid falling for products or practices that do not do what they claim.

---

1. "Peptides Are All the Same"

One big myth is that all peptides do the same thing. This likely comes from ads that talk about "the power of peptides" as if they are one single substance. In reality, there are countless possible peptide sequences, each with its own shape and function. Some peptides help with signals in the brain, some help build muscle, and others help with skin repair. A peptide that raises insulin levels in the blood is nothing like a peptide that helps skin hold moisture.

Peptide size also varies. Some have just two or three amino acids, while others have several dozen. The effect on the body depends on the exact sequence of amino acids, their arrangement, and how they interact with cells. This is why lumps of talk about "peptides" can be misleading. If someone tells you about "a peptide product" but does not name which peptide it contains, that is a red flag.

---

2. "Peptides Are a Recent Invention"

Another false idea is that peptides are a new discovery made by modern science. While laboratory technology has improved the ability to make and study peptides, nature has used them for ages. They exist in nearly all living things—bacteria, plants, and animals. They are part of the basic makeup of life. People have been aware of protein fragments and smaller chains for well over a century. Early scientists extracted them from tissues to see how they acted.

What changed over time is that we can now create synthetic peptides in labs with greater precision. We also have better tools to detect or measure them in samples. So the use of peptides in medicine or cosmetics may seem new, but the molecules themselves are not. When an advertisement calls them "breakthrough new molecules," it is partly ignoring the long history of these amino acid chains. The real breakthroughs involve figuring out how to apply peptides in more targeted ways.

---

3. "Peptides Are Magical Fixes"

Because peptides are linked to important signals or processes in the body, some people make bold claims that peptides can fix nearly anything. You might see products claiming to erase all wrinkles overnight, make hair grow inches in days, or help people lose huge amounts of weight without changing anything else. These kinds of promises are unrealistic. While certain peptides do show benefits, they are not miracle substances that can override natural limits or basic biology.

Real changes in the body—like improving skin texture or losing weight—generally come from a mix of factors such as diet, exercise, rest, and sometimes medical help. A peptide can assist in one part of the process, like signaling collagen growth or helping regulate appetite. But it is not a wand that solves every health or beauty challenge instantly. It is best to see peptides as helpful tools, not magic answers that remove the need for healthy habits.

---

4. "Peptides Only Help Bodybuilders and Athletes"

Peptides gained attention in sports for their possible roles in muscle growth or recovery. Some athletes misused them to try to gain an unfair edge, causing a lot of talk about doping. As a result, many people now think peptides are only for those who want bigger muscles or faster race times. In truth, peptides are used in many ways that do not involve extreme sports performance.

For example, doctors prescribe certain peptides to help regulate blood sugar. Some are used in skincare to help with dryness or fine lines. Others may help with wound repair or stress management. Everyday tasks in the body rely on peptides, from the immune system to digestion. So while some peptides are indeed of interest to athletes, they are only a small slice of the wide spectrum of how these molecules function.

---

5. "If It Says 'Peptide' on the Label, It Must Work"

Sometimes, a product has "peptides" in its ingredients and people think it must be effective. Marketers may add a tiny bit of a peptide to a cream or serum just to list it on the label, hoping it will catch attention. However, many factors decide if that product actually helps. These factors include:

1. **Type of Peptide**: Which specific sequence is being used? Is it the right one for the intended effect?
2. **Concentration**: Is there enough peptide included to do anything meaningful, or is it just a trace amount?
3. **Stability**: Can the peptide remain active in the product's formula? Some peptides break down if the pH is not right or if the container is not well-sealed.
4. **Delivery Method**: If a cream is supposed to target deeper layers, does it have the means to help the peptide get there?

An honest brand will often provide more data about the peptide and how much they are using. They might share the test results or references to studies on that peptide. If a label just says "peptides" with no specifics and no explanation, you might doubt how beneficial the product really is.

---

6. "Only Synthetic Peptides Matter"

There is a belief that natural peptides from plants or foods are useless compared to lab-made versions. In some circles, it is the other way around, with people claiming only "natural peptides" do any good. The fact is, both synthetic and natural peptides can be beneficial. Synthetic peptides are easier to tailor, changing single amino acids to improve stability or targeting. Natural peptides come with a history of being produced by living organisms, so we might find helpful ones that evolution has already shaped.

What truly matters is the structure and function of the peptide, not just where it comes from. Synthetic peptides can be more focused for medical uses, but they might be more expensive. Natural peptides in foods may be helpful to health, but they are often digested, so their direct effects can be smaller or less direct. People who claim only one source is valid might be oversimplifying things.

---

7. "Peptide Supplements Work Immediately"

Many supplement ads suggest that taking a peptide pill or powder will bring fast results, such as more energy or less joint pain within hours. In reality, the body does not usually respond that quickly. A swallowed peptide might be broken down in the stomach and intestines, turning into smaller fragments or single amino acids. Some might survive to have an effect, but it may take days or weeks of regular intake to see any noticeable results—if they occur at all.

It is also possible that a peptide must accumulate or trigger changes that only become clear over time. For example, a collagen peptide product aimed at the skin could take several weeks to affect how skin looks. Quick changes might be from something else in the product, like stimulants or a big dose of vitamins. But that is different from the action of the peptide itself. So if a supplement claims "overnight success," you can suspect that might be an exaggeration.

---

8. "More Peptides Means More Benefits"

Some people think that if a product has many different peptides, it must be better. Or that taking very high doses of a single peptide will amplify the effect without limit. Biological systems do not always work this way. The body needs specific signals in the right amounts. Sending too many signals at once or overloading a pathway can lead to confusion or side effects. It is like pressing all the buttons on a machine hoping it will run better, but in fact, it might break.

In skincare, stacking multiple peptide serums can be counterproductive if they have competing actions or if the formulas are not designed to work together. In medical settings, a doctor usually prescribes a specific dose for a reason. Going beyond that dose can cause unwanted effects on blood pressure, hormone levels, or metabolism. Balanced use—guided by evidence—is generally safer than the "more is better" approach.

9. "Topical Peptides Always Penetrate Deeply"

Skincare products sometimes claim that peptides in a lotion will reach deep skin layers or even the bloodstream. But the outer layer of the skin, called the stratum corneum, is very good at blocking substances. Peptides, which can be fairly large molecules, do not easily pass through unless the formula has special techniques (like certain delivery agents or smaller, modified peptide fragments).

Some peptides in creams act on the outermost cells and might help smooth or hydrate the surface. Others may prompt mild improvements by signaling just beneath the surface. However, if a brand says it can "deliver peptides right into your bloodstream through a simple rub," that is likely not accurate. Specialized methods—like patches or micro-needling—may help some ingredients move deeper, but standard creams have limited depth. This does not make them useless, but it does mean we should be realistic about how far they can go.

10. "Peptides Are Always Safe and Risk-Free"

Many peptides do come from natural processes in the body, making people assume they have no potential harm. But "natural" does not always mean zero risks. If a peptide affects the balance of hormones, blood sugar, or other systems, it can create problems if misused. For instance, a peptide that raises growth hormone might help in certain medical cases, but at excessive doses or in the wrong person, it can strain organs or cause abnormal tissue growth.

Even topical peptides can cause skin irritation or allergic reactions in some people. The chance may be small, but it is not zero. This does not mean peptides are dangerous in general—many are quite mild. It only means that they should be used with understanding and caution, as with any active ingredient. Thinking of them as totally harmless can lead to unexpected issues if users do not follow guidelines.

11. "You Must Inject All Peptides to Get Any Benefit"

In some areas, peptides are associated with injections, especially in sports. This leads to the idea that you can only get results if you inject them. In fact, the method of use depends on the peptide and what it is supposed to do. Some medical peptides must be injected because the digestive system would break them down otherwise, or because they need to get into the bloodstream directly. Others can be given as nasal sprays, patches, or creams that target local areas.

Some dietary peptides, like certain collagen fragments, are swallowed and might aid the body indirectly by providing amino acids or triggering minor signals in the gut. The results can be more subtle or slower than an injected peptide that floods the bloodstream, but it is still a possible route. So while injections are common for specific medical uses, not all peptide-based approaches require a needle.

---

12. "Peptides Replace the Need for a Healthy Lifestyle"

A tempting myth is that if you use the "right" peptides, you can ignore diet, activity, or other healthy habits. This has never been shown to be true. For instance, a peptide that regulates appetite might help you feel full sooner, but if you consistently eat junk foods in large portions, it may not lead to lasting weight control. A peptide that helps with muscle repair can make workouts more effective, but you still have to do the exercise.

The body's overall condition arises from sleep, stress levels, genetics, daily diet, physical activity, and more. Peptides can assist or fine-tune certain signals, but they do not override everything else. Good sleep alone might do more for hormone balance and recovery than a mild peptide supplement. People who treat peptides as an addition to healthy routines often see better outcomes than those who expect peptides to do all the work.

---

13. "Using Peptides Means You Are Doping"

In sports, doping refers to using banned substances that give unfair advantages. Some peptides, such as those that mimic growth hormones, are banned in professional competitions. But many peptides are not on banned lists and are used legally in beauty products or medical treatments. A person might use a peptide-based skin serum or take certain dietary peptides for joint health without any link to doping.

Confusion arises when people see news stories about athletes caught taking certain injected peptides. That does not mean all peptides are doping agents. It simply means some types that alter performance are banned. Each sports organization has a specific list of substances to avoid. People outside competitive sports do not automatically break doping rules by using a cosmetic peptide or a prescription peptide under a doctor's supervision.

14. "Peptides Are Too Fragile to Be Effective"

Because peptides can break down in heat, acid, or certain enzymes, some think they cannot work once outside the body's normal conditions. It is true that you must handle them carefully. Many peptides must be stored in a cool place or in special packaging. If they are in a cream, the formula might be designed to keep them stable. If they are in a supplement, they might be coated to survive the stomach.

Though peptides are somewhat delicate, modern manufacturing and formulation techniques allow them to remain active long enough to help. Stabilizing groups or special coatings can protect them from early breakdown. So it is not correct to say they are all "too fragile." You just have to look for products or prescriptions that have addressed this stability issue properly.

15. "You Can't Find Peptides in Everyday Foods"

Some people think peptides only come from labs or fancy products, so they believe normal diets do not contain them. But anytime we eat protein, it gets broken down into peptides and amino acids as part of digestion. Various food items naturally contain shorter peptide chains. For instance, aged cheese, fermented soy, and even some grains may have peptides released by enzymes or microbes.

Of course, these dietary peptides may not act in the same way as a carefully designed medical peptide. Often, they get broken down further or pass into the bloodstream in small amounts. But that does not mean they are absent from common meals. In fact, some of these peptides might have small positive effects, such as supporting heart health or modulating blood pressure. A balanced diet can provide a variety of these naturally occurring peptides.

---

16. "If It Works for Someone Else, It Will Work for You"

Testimonials about peptide-based products often appear online, showing how well they worked for one person. That can lead others to think they will have the exact same experience. The body's response to a peptide can vary widely due to differences in genetics, lifestyle, health status, and more. A person who sees big improvement in skin quality might have had a particular deficiency that the peptide helped. Another person might not have that same deficiency or might have other limiting factors.

This does not mean that anecdotes are always false. But they are not guaranteed results. A more reliable sign is when multiple studies or clinical trials show a consistent effect for a wide range of people, along with details about who benefits most. If someone says, "It helped me lose weight in a week," that does not prove it will do the same for anyone else. Good science involves bigger groups and consistent findings.

---

17. "All Collagen Peptides Are Created Equal"

Collagen peptides get a lot of buzz in the beauty and supplement world. Some think that any collagen powder will improve hair, skin, or nails identically. In truth, the source (fish, bovine, chicken, etc.), the processing method, and the size of the peptide fragments can all affect how they behave. Studies on certain collagen peptides show improvements in skin elasticity or joint comfort, but not all brands produce the same types or quality.

Some products may be mostly filler with minimal active collagen peptides. Others might have a different molecular weight that does not match what certain studies tested. The result is that "collagen peptide" can mean many things. Consumers who want real evidence should look for brands referencing actual research on that specific form of collagen peptide, not just random collagen claims.

18. "Peptides Give Quick Results for Aging Skin"

Because many skin creams advertise peptides, people may expect instant changes—like deep wrinkles vanishing in a few days. But healthy skin repair and collagen building take time. A peptide-based cream might help prompt cells in the skin to produce more structural proteins, but that is a slow process. It might take weeks or months of consistent use to see a moderate difference.

Any product that shows a quick effect is likely relying on temporary plumpers, silicone-based smoothing, or reflective particles that hide lines. That can be a nice cosmetic effect, but it is not the same as truly boosting collagen in deeper layers. Real improvements in skin density or elasticity need patience, consistent care, and avoidance of damaging factors like too much sun.

19. "Peptides Don't Need Regulation"

Some people argue that since peptides are naturally found in the body, they should not be regulated. But the truth is that unsafe or dishonest products can still emerge, especially when making synthetic peptides or combining them in new formulas. If a peptide claims to treat diseases or cause strong bodily changes, it might be regulated as a drug. If it is in a cream or a supplement, it should still meet safety rules and proper labeling requirements.

Regulation helps ensure that what is on the label matches what is in the container, and that the product is not harmful. Without oversight, some products might contain contaminants, or they might make unfounded health claims. Proper regulation does not stifle peptides; it helps them be used responsibly and fairly.

20. Moving Beyond the Myths

Peptides carry great potential in areas like medicine, beauty, and general wellness, but they are also subject to a lot of hype and misunderstandings. By looking at these myths in detail, we see that peptides are not a single, uniform substance, nor are they cures for everything. They can help in targeted ways when made and used properly, but their effects are typically gradual and must fit into a broader context of healthy living or medical guidance.

The best approach is to be informed. Check which specific peptide a product contains, see if there are credible studies behind it, and be realistic about results. Recognize that each person's body is unique, and that peptides, while valuable, are only part of the overall picture of health or skin care. With this balanced view, you can keep the good parts of what peptides offer without falling for myths that promise too much or ignore how biology truly works.

Chapter 16: Natural Sources of Peptides

When people think of peptides, they might picture high-tech labs or synthetic formulas. But nature has been making peptides forever. Plants and animals rely on them for many tasks, like defense, growth, and signals between cells. Humans often consume or encounter peptides in daily life without even noticing. In this chapter, we will explore natural places where peptides arise, how they are formed, and what benefits they may have. We will also discuss how cooking or processing affects them and whether you can get useful amounts of peptides simply by eating certain foods.

---

1. Peptides in Everyday Foods

Protein-rich foods like meat, fish, eggs, and dairy contain long amino acid chains. During digestion, enzymes break these proteins into smaller pieces—amino acids and peptides. Some of these peptides might be absorbed into the bloodstream before being broken down completely. Others might do their work within the gut itself, influencing signals related to appetite or gut health.

1. **Dairy**: Milk proteins, such as casein and whey, can produce bioactive peptides when they are partially digested or fermented. Some of these peptides might help with calcium absorption or mild blood pressure support.
2. **Soy Products**: Soy protein is known for releasing small chains that may have benefits like lowering certain markers of blood pressure or supporting cholesterol balance.
3. **Meat and Fish**: The proteins in these foods can break down into peptides that could help in muscle support or other bodily processes, although the effects are usually smaller than direct medical peptides.
4. **Legumes and Seeds**: Beans, lentils, and some seeds contain protein that is converted into peptides during cooking or fermentation. Certain peptides may have antioxidant or other helpful properties.

These dietary peptides are a natural part of eating complete proteins. While they do not always act as powerfully as specially designed therapeutic peptides, they show that normal meals can provide more than just basic nutrients.

2. Fermented Foods and Peptide Formation

Fermented foods are a special case for natural peptides. Microbes break down proteins, creating shorter chains that might not appear in fresh versions of the food. Examples include yogurt, kefir, cheese, miso, tempeh, and certain fermented vegetables. During fermentation, enzymes from bacteria or fungi snip proteins into smaller peptides.

Some of these peptides may have interesting effects. For instance, certain fermented dairy products contain peptides thought to ease blood vessel tension, possibly helping with blood pressure balance. Meanwhile, miso or soy sauce can have peptides that add savory flavor (umami) along with potential health benefits. Scientists are still unraveling exactly how these peptides act in the human body, since the digestive system can break them down further. Still, fermented foods remain an ancient and natural way to generate peptide-rich meals.

---

3. Plants That Use Peptides for Defense

In nature, plants cannot run from threats, so they develop chemical defenses. Some plants produce small peptides that deter insects or fight off fungi and bacteria. These defensive peptides might punch holes in a pest's cells or disrupt the pest's digestion. While these plant peptides are mainly for the plant's own protection, scientists study them to see if they could help people. Some labs test whether these peptides could become new antimicrobial agents or preservatives.

A few examples:

- **Potatoes** have small peptides that discourage insects from feeding on them.
- **Tomatoes** and other nightshade plants can produce peptides that warn pests to stay away.
- **Seeds** of certain grains carry peptides that protect them from mold growth.

We usually do not notice these defensive peptides while eating plants because they are in low concentrations, or they may be broken down during cooking. Nonetheless, they show how common peptides are in the living world.

4. Marine Organisms and Unique Peptides

Oceans hold many creatures that produce unusual peptides. Sponges, corals, and other sea life often make chemical compounds to defend themselves or to communicate. Because marine environments can be harsh, these organisms evolve potent molecules that help them survive. For instance, certain peptides from marine sources can block viruses or kill harmful bacteria without hurting the host. Researchers look into these marine peptides to see if they can be adapted for medicines.

Marine organisms might also have peptides that help cells handle high salt levels or changes in pressure. Scientists are curious whether these could be harnessed to protect human tissues, though this is still an emerging area. Some peptides discovered in sponges or tunicates might turn out to be useful leads for new drugs. Much remains to be studied, but the variety of marine life makes it a treasure chest for finding unique peptide structures.

5. Honeybees, Wasps, and Other Insects

Insects and other small animals also use peptides. Honeybees produce royal jelly that contains small protein fragments. Bees and wasps create venom with peptides that can shock or harm predators. Although venom is often painful for humans, it can yield chemicals that might be turned into medication. For example, some venom peptides may reduce swelling or affect nerve signals in a precise way.

Studies on insect-based peptides are still not widespread, but some labs have tested whether certain insect peptides could help fight bacteria or viruses. Because insects deal with many pathogens, their peptides might have protective roles that we can learn from. This does not mean people should start collecting insect venom at home—these are specialized cases for trained researchers who isolate and test exact compounds under safe conditions.

6. Why Natural Peptides Matter

Knowing where peptides appear in nature helps scientists see how life relies on these small chains. It also hints at how we might harness them for human benefit. Sometimes, a natural peptide discovered in a plant or microbe is later produced in a synthetic way for easier use. This merges the best of both worlds: a structure evolved by nature, combined with lab methods to make it in large amounts.

Natural peptides can also guide new ideas in drug design. For instance, if a plant peptide fights off fungi effectively, a modified version might help humans overcome fungal infections. If a marine creature produces a peptide that binds to a certain receptor, that might open the door for new treatments in humans who have faulty versions of that receptor. Researchers gather data from many organisms to see what might be applied more broadly.

---

7. Cooking and Processing: Effects on Peptides

How we prepare food can change the peptides inside it. High heat can unfold proteins and break them into fragments. Enzymes in marinating solutions can also generate new peptides. Fermentation, as noted, can yield a range of shorter chains. In many cases, cooking creates simpler peptides from bigger proteins, potentially making some foods easier to digest.

On the other hand, if heat is too intense or cooking is too long, the newly formed peptides might be destroyed further. Boiling, frying, baking—all can shift the breakdown pattern of proteins. This is neither entirely good nor entirely bad; it depends on which peptides are formed or lost. For people hoping to get certain special peptides in food, gentle cooking or partial fermentation might preserve them better than harsh processing.

---

8. Can Eating Peptides Help Health Directly?

Some consumers wonder if simply eating more natural peptide sources can bring medical-like benefits, such as lowering blood pressure or improving immunity. While studies show that specific food peptides may have mild positive effects, they are usually not as strong as a prescription drug. The main reason is that the digestive system is designed to break down and absorb proteins and peptides for general nutrition, not to deliver them in a targeted way to tissues.

However, a healthy diet that includes diverse protein sources may indeed provide small advantages over time. People who eat fermented foods, beans, dairy, fish, and more get a range of different peptides. While no single meal is likely to cause a dramatic effect, the long-term pattern could support well-being. It is best to think of dietary peptides as part of balanced nutrition rather than as a substitute for medical treatment.

9. Traditional Practices That Use Natural Peptides

Across different cultures, traditional foods or methods might increase the production or intake of peptides. For example:

- **Bone Broth**: Simmering bones for hours can break down collagen into gelatin and smaller peptides. Some people feel this broth helps with joint comfort or digestion.
- **Cheese Making**: Aging cheese lets enzymes work on milk proteins, generating flavor-rich peptides. Some aged cheeses are known to have peptides that might help with mild relaxation or blood vessel health.
- **Fermented Soy (Natto, Tempeh)**: Popular in certain parts of Asia, these dishes contain peptides formed by microbial fermentation. Some research hints they might help the body maintain normal blood clotting or other aspects of health.
- **Sourdough Bread**: The fermentation process can free peptides from wheat proteins, improving digestibility for some individuals.

While these cultural foods were developed for taste and preservation, the peptides they produce are an added benefit. Modern science is just catching up to the idea that these food traditions also involve complex chemistry.

10. The Line Between Natural and Synthetic

Sometimes, a peptide discovered in nature is synthesized in a lab. This might lead people to argue over whether it is still "natural." The chemical makeup is the same, but the production method is different. For people who like natural sources, the idea of a lab-synthesized product might feel less appealing. Meanwhile, synthetic production can offer higher purity or more consistent supply.

In many cases, it is not practical to harvest large amounts of a rare plant or marine creature to obtain a certain peptide. It may harm the environment or be too costly. That is why scientists prefer to copy the structure in the lab. The final molecule is chemically equivalent, even though the process is artificial. So a "natural" source can lead to a "synthetic" product that is still identical in function.

---

11. Challenges of Gathering Peptides from Wild Sources

Collecting peptides directly from wild plants or animals often poses ethical or environmental problems. If the species is rare or the process of extraction requires cutting down habitats, that is not sustainable. Also, the yield of the desired peptide may be tiny, meaning a lot of material must be used to get a small amount. Overharvesting can damage ecosystems.

Because of these difficulties, many scientists prefer to identify the structure of a promising natural peptide, then produce it with chemical synthesis or by using genetically modified microbes that can make it in a controlled setting. This way, we do not have to rely on large-scale harvesting from the wild. It is a safer approach for the environment and can produce a reliable supply of the peptide for research or commercial use.

---

12. Homemade Preparations for Peptide Benefits

Some people try to create "peptide-rich" recipes or homemade extracts. For instance, they might soak certain beans for a long time, then blend them, hoping to release beneficial peptides. Or they might brew long-simmered soups with bones or fish heads. While these efforts might produce small amounts of certain peptides, it is tough to measure or confirm which ones are present. The taste and smell also factor in—some processes that release peptides can result in strong odors if not done carefully.

If you enjoy traditional bone broth or fermented foods, that might be a pleasant addition to your diet. Just understand it is not guaranteed to mimic a targeted peptide supplement. The best approach is simply to keep a balanced menu with a variety of protein sources and consider including some fermented items. This way, you naturally get a spread of these tiny chains without having to worry about lab testing.

13. Do Natural Peptides Have Fewer Side Effects?

A claim you might see is that natural peptides are gentler or safer than synthetic peptides. This is not always true. The shape and action of a peptide matter more than whether it came from a lab or a plant. For example, certain plant peptides can be toxic to insects—and might harm human cells if taken in large amounts. On the other hand, a synthetic peptide designed for therapy could be safer if it specifically targets only one receptor.

In daily foods, peptides are often present in low amounts, and they have been part of human diets for centuries, so we know they are generally safe in those forms. Problems could arise if someone isolates a natural peptide in a high concentration and misuses it. So there is nothing automatically safer about natural peptides, though common foods containing them tend to pose little risk for most healthy people.

14. The Role of Microbes in Our Gut

One reason dietary peptides might still matter is the microbiome. Our gut is home to many microbes that continue breaking down proteins after we eat. They can free more peptides that might then influence gut health or immune responses. This area of research is growing quickly, as scientists uncover how microbe-made peptides (or microbes helping release peptides from food) could impact overall wellness.

If a certain bacterium in the gut excels at forming a beneficial peptide from a protein you eat, that might help your body in ways we do not fully understand yet. People have different microbiomes, so the same meal could yield different peptide results in different individuals. This is one reason why some people respond better to certain diets than others. The synergy between dietary proteins, microbial enzymes, and the body's own processes is very intricate.

15. Finding Natural Peptide Supplements

Some companies sell "natural peptide extracts" from sources like fish collagen or certain plant seeds. They often highlight that these are "not synthetic" and claim broad benefits. While fish collagen is widely used in beauty supplements, the user experience can vary. Some might notice improvements in hair or skin, while others see less effect. The differences could be due to how each person's body processes the peptides or how consistent they are with their routine.

When picking a natural peptide supplement, consider:

- **Source**: Is it from fish, bovine, or another origin? Do you have allergies to that source?
- **Processing Method**: Is it hydrolyzed or partially broken down? That might improve absorption.
- **Purity**: Are there any tests for heavy metals or contaminants (especially in marine products)?
- **Company Reputation**: Do they share data on how they prepare and verify the peptides?

These points help you choose more wisely if you decide to try a natural peptide supplement.

16. Are Insect or Worm Protein Powders Rich in Peptides?

As the global demand for protein grows, some look to insects or worms as alternative protein sources. When these proteins are processed, do they yield interesting peptides? Possibly. Insects have a variety of amino acid sequences, and partial digestion or fermentation might free some peptides. But research is still early. People who use insect-based flour or meal might simply be aiming for a high-protein, eco-friendly food. Any peptide benefits beyond that would be a bonus, not a well-documented fact yet.

17. Natural Peptide Research in Farms and Agriculture

Peptides do not just show up in foods for human meals. Farmers also use them in animal feed or in protecting crops. For example, certain antimicrobial peptides can shield plants from pests or infections. In livestock, adding small peptide supplements might help animals use nutrients more efficiently, though that practice must be checked for safety and any effects on meat or milk. This area is part of a push to reduce antibiotics by using more targeted approaches that rely on nature's own weapons against disease.

---

18. Possible Future Directions

As we learn more about natural peptides, we may see:

1. **Selective Breeding**: Farmers might choose plant strains that produce more beneficial peptides, or that break down into these peptides after harvest.
2. **Tailored Fermentation**: Companies might design special fermentation methods to create foods with targeted peptides for digestion or mild health support.
3. **Eco-Friendly Bio-Pesticides**: Natural peptides from plants or insects could become safer alternatives to chemical pesticides, reducing harm to the environment.
4. **Medicinal Adaptations**: Peptides found in rare marine species might inspire new classes of drugs for infections, inflammation, or other conditions.

These possibilities rely on deeper knowledge of how peptides behave in nature and how we can apply them responsibly.

---

19. Appreciating the Simplicity of Daily Foods

While it is exciting to hear about advanced uses of peptides, there is also value in recognizing that everyday meals already involve them. Eating balanced proteins from plant or animal sources, including fermented or aged options, can deliver a range of small peptides. Though the direct impact on health might be subtle, over a lifetime it could add up.

This is a reminder that basic nutrition, the way people have eaten for centuries—fresh foods, some fermentation, varied sources—has its own quiet complexity. Natural peptides are part of that story, working in the background to support bodily processes.

---

20. Conclusion: Embracing Nature's Peptide Wealth

Peptides occur throughout nature, from the foods on our plates to the sea creatures in the deep ocean. Plants and animals rely on them for growth, defense, and communication. By eating a variety of protein sources, including fermented or gently processed items, humans naturally consume small amounts of these chains. While they will not replace medical treatments or engineered peptide therapies for specific conditions, they do highlight how closely we are tied to these molecules every day.

Scientists continue to explore the vast library of peptides offered by nature. Some might lead to new solutions for fighting germs or healing tissues. Others might find a place in eco-friendly agriculture or specialized products. Meanwhile, the rest of us can see that peptides are not just high-tech inventions—they are part of life's basic building blocks, present all around us in the natural world.

Chapter 17: Future Prospects in Peptide Science

Peptides have grown from a niche area in research to a broad field touching medicine, cosmetics, food science, and more. Researchers worldwide keep looking for new ways to use these small amino acid chains, hoping they can solve problems where other solutions fall short. In this chapter, we will explore how peptide science might progress in the years to come. We will look at new tools, possible breakthroughs, and the steps needed for peptides to reach their full potential in various fields.

---

1. Expanding Roles in Medicine

Many experts see peptides as promising for treating illnesses that are hard to manage. Medications based on peptides can be designed to latch onto certain cells or signals in the body, making them precise and possibly safer than some older drugs. As technology improves, researchers can design peptides that resist breakdown or target organs more accurately. This precision may reduce side effects and allow for smaller doses.

We can expect more peptide therapies for conditions like:

- **Cancer**: Using peptides to guide drugs or the immune system to tumor cells.
- **Metabolic Disorders**: Improving blood sugar control or body weight management with advanced peptide formulas.
- **Autoimmune Issues**: Fine-tuning immune responses so the body does not attack its own tissues.
- **Chronic Inflammation**: Blocking harmful signals that cause ongoing swelling in joints or organs.

Some of these ideas have been tested in small trials. As time goes on, researchers hope to confirm that peptides can deliver consistent benefits without causing new problems.

---

2. Personalized Peptide Treatments

A key area of growth is personalized medicine, which matches a treatment to a person's unique biological makeup. Because peptides are short chains that can be made in many specific forms, they might be well-suited for this approach. For instance, if a tumor has a special marker, a lab can make a peptide that sticks only to that marker. If a patient has a certain genetic change affecting hormone signals, a peptide drug could be built to fix that signal.

Some companies are already testing personalized vaccines for cancer that include peptide fragments from a patient's tumor. The goal is to teach the immune system to attack cells carrying those fragments. This is still experimental, but if it works, it might shift how we see cancer care. Instead of a single drug for everyone, doctors might use tailored peptide vaccines or therapies.

---

3. Smarter Delivery Systems

Peptides are often fragile and can be destroyed by stomach acids or enzymes. That is why many peptide-based therapies come as injections. But not everyone wants regular shots. Looking ahead, scientists are testing delivery methods that protect peptides until they arrive at their target. Possible tactics include:

- **Nasal Sprays**: Letting peptides enter through the nose, bypassing some barriers.
- **Skin Patches**: Releasing peptides slowly through the skin.
- **Capsules with Coatings**: Special shells that survive stomach acid, dissolving only in certain parts of the gut.
- **Nanoparticle Carriers**: Tiny particles that shield peptides from breakdown and guide them to specific tissues.

If these approaches succeed, peptide treatments might become more convenient and less painful. This could open the door for more everyday uses, rather than limiting peptides mainly to hospitals or clinics.

4. Combining Peptides with Other Tech

Another likely path is pairing peptides with tools like nanotech or gene editing. Peptides can act as guides, steering nanoparticles to the right cells. Once there, the nanoparticle might drop off other drugs or even gene-editing tools like CRISPR components. This joined method could help fix or remove damaged genes without affecting healthy cells.

Scientists also talk about "peptide scaffolds," where a peptide-based framework supports cells in growing new tissue. If you have an injured part of the body, a scaffold might help cells rebuild by giving them a structure to fill in. Over time, the body replaces the scaffold with natural tissue. This concept is still being tested but might lead to better healing for bone breaks or organ damage.

---

5. New Peptides from Computation

Thanks to stronger computers, we can use software to predict how a protein or peptide will fold. We can also guess how it might bind to a receptor. Researchers feed the computer a target shape and ask it to create a peptide that fits that shape well. This "in silico" (computer-based) design can speed up discovery because it avoids random lab tests. Once the computer proposes a few sequences, scientists make them in the lab to confirm which works best.

As these programs improve, the time from an idea to a ready-to-test peptide may shrink. This could lead to a surge of new peptides for different purposes—fighting germs, balancing hormones, or calming overactive immune responses, among others. Quicker design cycles might also reduce costs, since fewer lab trials are wasted.

---

6. Sustainable and Eco-Friendly Production

Traditional peptide synthesis can use a lot of chemicals, leading to waste. The future likely involves finding greener ways to produce peptides. Some labs already explore:

- **Enzyme-Based Methods**: Using enzymes to link amino acids in water-based systems, cutting down on harsh solvents.
- **Microbial Factories**: Inserting genes into yeast or bacteria so they make the desired peptide naturally.
- **Continuous-Flow Reactors**: Automating the process in a single flow rather than many separate steps, reducing resource use.

As public interest in eco-friendly products grows, companies that adopt cleaner manufacturing might stand out. This could encourage broader change in the industry. Over time, if greener methods become cheaper and more reliable, they might replace many older synthesis practices.

7. Peptides in Everyday Healthcare

At present, many peptide drugs are used for specific cases, like insulin for blood sugar or certain hormones for growth problems. In the future, peptides might be part of normal healthcare for many conditions. For example, a person struggling with mild stress might be prescribed a safe, peptide-based nasal spray to help calm the body's signals. Someone with a stubborn infection might receive a short course of peptide antibiotics that target bacteria without harming beneficial microbes.

This shift depends on more research and acceptance by doctors and regulatory groups. Still, as we gain experience with peptides, it might become easier to approve them for everyday use. Advances in stability and cost-cutting also matter, because if a peptide treatment is too pricey or awkward to store, it may not catch on widely.

8. Peptide Vaccines Beyond Infectious Disease

Vaccines typically prime the immune system to recognize part of a virus or bacterium. Peptide-based vaccines do this by including short stretches of protein found in the invader. Right now, peptide vaccines for certain diseases are in development, and some have been tested in limited trials. The advantage is that peptides can be made very cleanly, reducing some side effects linked to whole-virus vaccines. They can also be tweaked to avoid parts of a virus that change often.

Beyond infections, the idea of a vaccine for non-infectious problems—like certain tumors or even chronic conditions—might expand. The immune system could be taught to remove harmful cells or proteins. If scientists learn to pick the right peptide segments that trigger a helpful immune response, we might see more advanced peptide-based vaccines hitting the market.

9. New Paths for Beauty and Skincare

Peptides are already in many skin products. Future lines could be more advanced, with formulas that deliver peptides deeper, or that combine different peptides for a stronger effect. Imagine a serum that uses a stable peptide to reduce redness, another to help collagen, and another to keep hydration levels balanced—all carefully protected so they do not break down quickly. We might also see "smart" cosmetics that respond to changes in skin pH or temperature, releasing peptides only when needed.

Some companies may also test if peptides can help scalp health and hair growth more reliably. Current products often rely on anecdotal reports. In the future, we might have well-studied peptides that genuinely strengthen hair follicles or reduce hair loss, validated by scientific data rather than just marketing.

10. Peptide Foods and Functional Nutrition

People already buy collagen peptide powders to stir into drinks or foods. Moving forward, we may see more foods enriched with specific peptides to help with minor health goals, like supporting joint function or mild stress control. The main challenge is proving that ingesting these peptides leads to consistent benefits in the real world, since digestion can break many of them down.

Another angle is using peptides in natural food preservation. If a certain peptide can fight bacteria on surfaces, it might prolong the shelf life of fresh foods. This could reduce waste without relying solely on chemical preservatives. Some food research labs test antimicrobial peptides from plants, hoping they can keep items like fresh produce safer for longer. If these tests succeed, you might see labels mentioning "naturally derived peptides" as a means of protection.

11. Peptide Sensors and Diagnostics

Peptides can bind to certain molecules with high precision. This property can be used in sensors to detect toxins, disease markers, or other targets. For instance, a test strip might have a peptide that changes color when it meets a specific virus protein. Healthcare workers could then quickly see if a sample contains that virus. Similar peptide-based diagnostic tools might be placed on surfaces to monitor water quality or food safety.

Though many of these concepts are still in labs, the potential is large. Peptide sensors might be cheaper and easier to produce than some antibody-based tests, and they could be stable if engineered correctly. We might see portable, peptide-based testing kits in clinics, homes, or workplaces. These could provide quick readings for things like infection risk, allergic substances, or even air quality factors.

12. Artificial Intelligence and Peptide Research

Artificial intelligence (AI) can search massive data sets faster than people can. It can spot patterns about how certain peptides fold or how they interact with cell receptors. AI might also predict how changes in a peptide's sequence alter its effect. Researchers can use these insights to pick the best candidates to make in the lab.

As big tech companies join in, or as specialized biotech firms adopt AI-driven methods, the speed of peptide discovery may rise sharply. This could lead to more personalized approaches, as AI sifts through a person's genetic profile to propose a custom peptide therapy. Of course, we are not there yet, but the foundation is being laid by ongoing projects.

13. Widening the Public View of Peptides

Right now, the average person might only connect peptides to sports doping or fancy skin creams. That public view could change if more peptide-based medicines appear. As doctors prescribe peptides for everyday ailments, and as people see them working in real life, general knowledge about peptides could improve.

Public outreach by scientists, clearer product labels, and media coverage might help more people see peptides as a normal, well-researched option, not an exotic or suspicious ingredient. Schools and museums might even include exhibits on how peptides work in the body, much like they do for DNA or vitamins. Better understanding can help people use peptide products responsibly and avoid falling for scams.

14. Addressing Cost and Access

A big question about peptide therapies is whether they will be affordable. Some are pricey to make, especially if they require advanced production. As research expands, methods might become cheaper. Large-scale factories or continuous-flow systems can boost efficiency. Also, if insurance plans see proven benefits, they might cover certain peptide-based treatments, making them more widely available.

Still, cost will remain a hurdle for a while. Low-income areas may not have easy access to the newest peptide options. Organizations that support global health will likely push for tech transfer to local manufacturers, or for licensing deals that let them produce key peptides at reduced prices. This has happened with some vaccines and medicines in the past, and it might happen with peptides too, ensuring that breakthroughs reach more people worldwide.

15. Ethical and Regulatory Questions

As peptides become more powerful, new ethical points could emerge. For example, if there is a peptide that safely boosts muscle growth, do we allow healthy people to use it, or do we limit it to medical needs? If a peptide changes social behavior (like an enhanced version of oxytocin), could that be misused? Regulators will have to decide where to set boundaries.

Strong oversight is important. We do not want to see a rush of unproven peptides that promise unrealistic gains. Regulators like the FDA or EMA will continue to require testing, but they also need to adapt to new research methods that produce peptides faster than before. They may adopt special frameworks to handle personalized or AI-designed peptides. Balancing safety with innovation will be a major ongoing task.

---

16. Collaboration Across Fields

Peptide science is not limited to chemistry or biology alone. It involves software engineers, medical doctors, food technologists, farmers, and environmental experts. An effective peptide that fights crop pests might need input from agricultural scientists, ecologists, and regulatory experts to be sure it does not harm helpful insects or the soil. A medical peptide for cancer might need large clinical trials, but also AI specialists to design and refine it, plus biotech firms to scale production.

This cross-field teamwork is growing. Universities and private labs often form partnerships, pooling their skills. Government grants may support big projects that combine multiple branches of science. International meetings on peptide science bring together groups that might otherwise never meet. In the future, more of these cooperative efforts can speed discoveries and help ensure that peptides are used responsibly.

---

17. Public Awareness of Risks and Rewards

While the future of peptide science sounds bright, it is important for the public to keep an even view. Peptides can do impressive things, but they have limits. They can also have side effects or be expensive. We might see unscrupulous sellers push fad peptide products with no real proof, hoping to exploit hype. Balanced news coverage and honest marketing are essential.

If you see claims like "Reverse aging overnight with the ultimate peptide" or "Eat this peptide to lose 10 pounds in a day," you can guess that it is marketing fluff. Real progress takes time. Real benefits often arrive in small steps, not radical leaps. Over the next decades, peptides could become a normal part of healthcare, but they will not make all other treatments vanish. Each condition might need a mix of solutions.

18. Training the Next Generation

To keep peptide science growing, schools and colleges will need to train students in the relevant fields—biochemistry, molecular biology, computational design, manufacturing, and more. As the job market for peptide-related work expands, teaching labs might offer courses on peptide synthesis, testing, and data analysis.

The next generation of researchers could combine lab skills with AI or specialized knowledge of a certain disease area. They may also learn about ethics and regulations early on, ensuring that future scientists think beyond the lab bench. Hands-on internships at biotech companies or research hospitals could give them real-world experiences. This well-rounded training is crucial if we want steady progress rather than random breakthroughs that stall due to lack of proper follow-up.

19. Possible Surprises

Science often brings unexpected turns. Peptides might surprise us in new ways, such as:

- **Quantum Biology Links**: Some researchers hint that peptide folding might connect to tiny quantum effects, though this is speculative.
- **Hybrid Molecules**: Merging peptides with synthetic polymers or metals to create unusual structures for electronics or smart materials.
- **Interplanetary Uses**: In the far future, if humans venture deeper into space, stable peptides that protect cells from radiation could be a niche, though it sounds like science fiction today.

While these ideas might seem far-off, the history of science is full of developments that started out as wild theories. The flexible nature of peptides means they could pop up in fields we do not even suspect yet.

20. Conclusion: A Landscape of Possibilities

Looking ahead, peptides seem set to play a larger role across medicine, food, environment, and more. Each step forward—like better stability, new delivery methods, or AI-driven design—opens fresh avenues. Yet real success will depend on careful research, fair regulations, and broad cooperation among experts. Costs and ethical guidelines must be tackled alongside the science itself.

In the end, peptides can enrich our options in many areas, from advanced cancer treatments to safer crop protection. They are not quick-fix answers to everything, but they do offer a flexible platform for innovation. As we learn more, the boundaries of what peptides can do may keep expanding. If guided well, the near future could see peptides become trusted helpers in daily health and beyond, supporting people in ways that once seemed out of reach.

Chapter 18: Ethics of Peptide Use

Science and technology can move swiftly, offering new ways to address health, beauty, and other concerns. As peptides expand into different sectors—medicine, skin care, sports, and beyond—it raises questions about fairness, safety, and social responsibility. Who should have access to certain peptides? How do we ensure that people do not use them in ways that harm themselves or others? Where do we draw the line between needed medical therapy and enhancement for personal gain? In this chapter, we will look at these ethical dilemmas, focusing on transparency, fairness, legal matters, and the impact on society.

1. Defining Ethical Use

Ethical use of peptides means using them in a way that respects human health, follows relevant laws, and considers how they affect society at large. It also involves being honest about what a peptide product can and cannot do. If a substance is intended to treat a real medical condition, that is different from using the same substance for non-medical reasons, such as chasing unrealistic body standards or attempting to gain an edge over others.

Peptides can blur lines because they come in so many forms and serve so many functions. A doctor might prescribe a peptide for a hormone imbalance, a lab might create a peptide that fights bacteria in crops, or a beauty brand might add a peptide to a face cream. Each of these examples has different ethical angles. Whenever a peptide can alter bodily processes, fairness and safety become points of concern.

2. Medical vs. Non-Medical Uses

Many peptide-based treatments arise from a need to help patients with real health problems. For instance, a person with low insulin production can use peptide therapies to help control blood sugar. A child with growth issues might receive growth hormone-related peptides under medical oversight. In these cases, it is not controversial, because the goal is to restore what the body lacks.

However, some people might want to use similar peptides for non-medical reasons. An adult could try to get the same hormone-based peptide simply to gain muscle mass or reduce body fat, even if there is no medical deficiency. This raises ethical debates. Should these substances be available for anyone seeking a shortcut to a more muscular body or to slow visible aging?

Supporters of expanded access argue that people should have the freedom to use peptides if they are informed of the risks. Opponents worry that misuse could lead to physical harm or a culture of constant enhancement, placing new pressures on those who do not want to use such methods. Regulators often set rules that limit the use of certain peptides to medical prescriptions, trying to steer them toward genuine health needs.

---

3. Fairness in Sports

Peptide use in sports is a well-known ethical topic. Professional athletes may look for substances that help them recover quickly or build muscle, creating a competitive advantage. Anti-doping agencies frequently ban many performance-enhancing peptides. The logic is that sports should measure natural ability plus training, not pharmacological boosts.

Yet doping remains a challenge because labs can be slow to detect new peptides. Athletes who can afford these cutting-edge therapies might cheat more easily. This undermines fairness. Even in amateur sports, some individuals try to use peptides to outperform their peers, which raises similar questions on a smaller scale.

When doping scandals break, public trust in sports can waver. Some fans believe that if advanced tools exist, maybe we should allow them, as long as they are safe. Others see that as undermining the spirit of honest competition. The key ethical point is about respecting equal chances for all. If peptides that boost performance are only available to wealthy or well-connected athletes, the playing field tilts. That is why doping rules remain strict, although policing them can be tricky.

---

4. Cosmetic Enhancement and Social Pressure

Beyond sports, peptides appear in beauty products to address skin concerns or hair problems. On the surface, this seems harmless. But it can get complex if society starts expecting everyone to use such enhancements. If peptides become a norm for looking youthful, people who cannot afford them or who prefer not to use them might face increased social pressure.

People have always sought ways to maintain or improve appearance, whether through makeup, hair dyes, or plastic surgery. Peptides add another layer because they can go deeper than surface products—they may alter cell signals related to collagen or hair follicles. Ethical questions arise: does widespread cosmetic peptide use push unrealistic beauty ideals? Does it create a market where people feel obligated to spend large sums on advanced products to "keep up"?

Some argue that each person should decide for themselves without moral judgment. Others worry about marketing hype that makes peptides sound essential for "anyone who cares about their skin," driving unrealistic expectations. Honesty in advertising and accessible pricing can help, but ethical lines remain fuzzy if peptides become a social requirement rather than an individual choice.

---

5. Access and Health Equity

Cost, insurance coverage, and distribution play major roles in who gets to benefit from peptide breakthroughs. Specialized peptide treatments can be very expensive, making them hard to obtain for those with lower income or limited health coverage. This creates disparities. If a new peptide therapy is the best option for a serious condition, but only wealthy patients can afford it, that raises fairness concerns.

Health organizations aim to manage such issues by negotiating prices or offering assistance programs. Sometimes, nonprofits or government bodies step in to subsidize life-saving peptides. However, for less critical conditions, public funding might not be as available. People living in remote regions might not have specialists who can prescribe or monitor peptide use.

An ethical approach tries to ensure that essential peptide-based treatments are not limited to privileged groups. It also involves balancing company profits with the moral duty to serve public health. Some critics see modern pharmaceuticals as placing profit above patient access, while industry members argue they need returns to fund research. Navigating this tension is part of the ethical puzzle in peptide use.

---

6. Transparency in Marketing and Labeling

Ethics also connect to how companies market and label peptide products. Ads might exaggerate benefits, skip over possible side effects, or remain vague about the actual peptide content. A jar of cream could list "peptides" as an ingredient but not identify which peptide or in what concentration. This leaves customers guessing and can lead to false hopes or wasted money.

An ethical approach to marketing would be upfront about:

- **Specific Peptides**: Naming which peptides are used (e.g., "Palmitoyl Tripeptide-1") rather than just saying "contains peptides."
- **Concentration**: Giving an approximate percentage so buyers know if it is a tiny sprinkle or a meaningful level.
- **Scientific Support**: Citing real studies or explaining the realistic timeline for results.
- **Possible Limitations**: Stating if the product is not suitable for certain skin types, or if the results might be mild and take time.

Regulatory agencies often require honesty, but enforcement can be uneven, especially for supplements or cosmetics. Ethical businesses adhere to clear labeling and avoid overpromising. This fosters trust and helps consumers make informed decisions. If a brand relies on vague claims like "will fix all aging problems," that is a red flag. Ethical standards suggest focusing on data and disclaimers, telling people what the product can realistically do.

---

7. Personal Responsibility vs. Societal Influence

One angle of ethics is deciding how much responsibility lies with the user, the seller, or the government. For instance, if a brand sells a peptide-based muscle enhancer that is not fully tested for safety, do we blame the company if users get hurt, or do we blame the users for taking the risk? If the brand claims "for research only" but markets to fitness communities, is that dishonest or is it up to users to heed the label?

Balancing personal freedom with consumer protection is a recurring theme. Some argue that adults should be able to choose what to do with their bodies. But others note that many people lack the medical background to gauge the real risks, especially with new peptides. That is why consumer protection laws exist—to stop misleading claims and reduce harm from shady products. However, black markets for peptides do thrive, especially online. This raises further questions about how to regulate globally and whether authorities can keep up with an ever-changing list of substances.

---

8. Environmental and Animal Considerations

Peptide production and use can also touch on environmental ethics. Factories that make peptides might release waste chemicals if they do not follow good manufacturing practices. Researchers gather peptides from marine sources or other organisms, risking ecological harm if done irresponsibly. Meanwhile, testing new peptides often involves animal studies. Scientists have tried to reduce animal use by shifting to cell-based tests, but it is not always possible to avoid live-animal trials, especially for safety.

Ethical guidelines encourage reducing environmental impact. They also promote the "3 Rs" in animal research: replace animal models where possible, reduce the number of animals used, and refine methods to minimize suffering. Some labs aim to create peptides from yeast or bacteria to avoid harvesting from wild ecosystems. Consumer choices can play a role, too: if people demand peptides from sustainable sources, manufacturers may adapt.

---

9. Cultural and Social Factors

Ethics intersect with cultural values. In some cultures, certain peptides might be linked to moral or religious concerns—for example, if they come from animal sources. Or there might be beliefs about altering the body with "unnatural" substances. People vary widely in how they view scientific interventions. A therapy that is common in one country might face pushback in another.

Global businesses must navigate these differences if they want acceptance. They may need to clarify whether a peptide is derived from pork, bovine, or synthetic routes. They might also need to respect local norms about body modification. This can be complicated, but ignoring it can lead to ethical conflicts and public backlash.

---

10. Children and Peptide Use

Using peptides in children's treatments brings extra scrutiny. If a child has a serious hormonal deficiency, peptides can be life-changing. But if parents or coaches start giving peptides to kids for athletic performance or faster growth, that is more controversial. Young bodies are still developing, and altering signals with peptides might have long-term consequences we do not fully understand.

Ethical pediatric care demands that any peptide therapy be guided by medical evidence. Doctors carefully weigh benefits against risks. Off-label or experimental use on children is a sensitive area. In many places, special rules govern clinical trials that include minors, requiring parental consent plus ethical review. If a child is old enough, they also need to understand and agree. This protects them from exploitation or from parents pushing them into questionable treatments.

---

11. Data Privacy and Genetic Links

As the field moves toward personalized peptides, labs might analyze a person's genes or health data to design custom treatments. This raises privacy issues. How securely are these genetic details stored? Who can see them? If private insurance companies gain access, might they discriminate based on the likelihood of needing certain peptide therapies?

Ethical guidelines push for anonymity, informed consent, and robust cybersecurity. People deserve to know how their genetic and health data will be used. They should have the right to say no to sharing it for commercial gain. If companies create a custom peptide for a patient, do they retain the right to sell that design to others with the same genetic profile? These questions do not have simple answers, but privacy protection is crucial for trust in the system.

---

12. Informed Consent

In both medical and research settings, informed consent is central. If you are given a peptide therapy, you should understand:

- **What the peptide is for**
- **Possible benefits and side effects**
- **Alternatives to this treatment**
- **Any uncertainties or experimental aspects**

Ethics demand that individuals freely choose whether to proceed, without feeling tricked or pressured. This goes beyond signing forms. Medical staff should explain in everyday language, encourage questions, and give people time to think it over. With new or experimental peptides, the unknowns may be greater, so it is even more important to be clear about risks.

For over-the-counter items, "consent" is less formal. Still, companies should offer enough information so buyers are not misled. If marketing is overly promotional, people cannot make a balanced decision. That can be seen as violating the spirit of informed consent.

---

13. Regulating Online Markets

A big ethical and legal challenge is the rise of online sales. Websites may sell peptides as "research chemicals" or "for lab use," but actually target bodybuilders, dieters, or others seeking quick fixes. This shadow market can skip safety testing, letting harmful or contaminated products spread. Authorities worldwide struggle to rein in these sellers, who might operate from countries with lax rules or change their websites often.

Some believe that tightening online restrictions or blocking certain key words might help, but it can also push trade further underground. Another approach is educating the public about the dangers of unverified peptides. People might be less tempted if they are aware that a big percentage of these online items are fake or impure. Better tracking, international collaboration, and severe penalties for major offenders might also curb the problem. But as technology advances, so do the methods of illegal vendors.

14. Balancing Innovation and Caution

Developing a new peptide can take years of lab work and trials. Some worry that too much caution delays treatments that patients need, while others say rushing brings bigger risks. Striking the right balance is hard. If regulators are too strict, research might slow and costs might rise. If they are too lenient, unsafe peptides might flood the market, harming public trust.

An ideal system supports high-quality research, ensures thorough testing, and speeds up approval for truly beneficial therapies, yet keeps unscrupulous claims in check. Some regions have "accelerated approval" pathways for drugs that address urgent health crises, but these can be misused if not carefully monitored. The tension between innovation and caution will keep shaping peptide policy.

15. Intellectual Property and Sharing Knowledge

Companies or labs can patent peptide sequences or production methods. This can lead to high prices for consumers if a firm has a monopoly. On the other side, patents encourage companies to invest in research. Without the chance to recoup costs, they might not fund expensive trials.

Some argue for open sharing of life-saving knowledge, especially for rare diseases or global health. Nonprofit groups sometimes push to waive patents, letting generic makers produce affordable peptides. Ethical questions arise: should we protect profits as a reward for innovation, or ensure widespread access to vital treatments? A balanced approach might include limited patents plus agreements for accessible pricing in lower-income regions. This approach has been seen in HIV drugs and might extend to peptide therapies if they become crucial for major diseases.

---

16. Potential Misuse and Black Markets

When peptides promise anti-aging, muscle gains, or weight control, black markets can emerge. People might be desperate for quick results or be lured by flashy claims. This can lead to organized crime involvement, unsafe production, and major health risks. Law enforcement alone cannot stop these markets if demand stays high. Education, open discussion of realistic expectations, and legitimate, safer channels for those who need peptides can reduce the appeal of illicit sources.

Another misuse scenario is weaponizing peptides as toxins. While it is unlikely for most peptides, some can harm cells or disrupt signals. There is a moral duty in the research community to watch for suspicious behavior or suspicious funding. Governments and institutions often have rules on "dual-use" research. They might classify certain peptides as controlled substances if they pose a security threat. Researchers should remain alert to how their work might be twisted and avoid collaborating with suspicious groups.

---

17. Ethical Use in Agriculture and Environment

Peptides are not only for humans. They can protect crops from pests or help animals grow faster. This might reduce chemical pesticides or antibiotics. But it can also lead to unintended ecological effects if not tested thoroughly. In agriculture, an ethical approach means ensuring that peptide-based pest controls do not harm beneficial insects or disrupt soil microbes.

For livestock, peptides that promote quick growth may bring the same concerns as hormone additives. Do they affect meat quality or animal welfare? Will consumers accept them if they think it is unnatural? Regulations may require thorough safety checks before allowing such practices. In addition, honest labeling is essential so people know how their food was produced. If farmland use of peptides spreads, balanced policies can help avoid repeating past mistakes with chemicals or antibiotics.

18. Moral Debates on Enhancement

One major ethical debate is enhancement vs. therapy. If a person's growth hormone is very low, a peptide might restore it to a normal range—that is therapy. But if a healthy person wants more muscle or wants to slow certain aspects of aging far beyond what is typical, that veers into enhancement territory. Opinions differ on whether that is acceptable. Some see it as personal choice. Others see a risk of pressuring everyone to join the "enhancement arms race."

Medical ethicists often discuss where normal health ends and enhancement begins. Peptides are tricky because they can do both. For instance, a small dose might treat a deficiency, while a higher dose might push the body beyond normal limits. If we allow open access, will we create a society where "natural" abilities are overshadowed by those who can buy better, faster, or stronger bodies? Or is that just an extension of technology we already accept, such as eyeglasses or prosthetics?

19. Building Ethical Frameworks

Given these issues, many groups are forming guidelines. For instance:

- **Professional Associations**: Doctors' or nurses' groups might advise members on prescribing peptides only for medically justified reasons.
- **Research Councils**: Scientific bodies could require ethics approval for certain peptide studies, focusing on risk and the potential for misuse.
- **Regulatory Agencies**: They decide which peptides need prescriptions, how they should be labeled, and which ones are banned in sports.
- **Public Discussion**: Workshops, debates, and articles can inform citizens about the pros and cons, gathering input before final rules are set.

When all these players share knowledge and weigh different views, the resulting policies are more likely to be balanced. Stakeholders can spot loopholes or identify undue burdens on certain groups. Without broad input, there is a risk of rules that either stifle valid research or let harmful practices slip by.

---

20. Conclusion: Moving Forward Responsibly

The rise of peptides offers real benefits in medicine, agriculture, and daily life. But to harness them wisely, we must address ethical questions head-on. That means ensuring fair access for medical needs, banning dangerous doping or false claims, and respecting each person's right to safe, accurate information. It also involves setting boundaries on enhancement and considering how a rush for "better" might create inequalities or health risks.

While no single approach will satisfy everyone, open dialogue and careful regulation can prevent extreme abuses. Scientists, doctors, companies, and the public share responsibility in shaping how we use peptides. By thinking about both the great potential and the real risks, we can keep the field on a path that benefits more people in the long run. The peptides themselves are neutral—they can help or harm, depending on our choices. Acting ethically ensures they become a positive force in health and beyond.

Chapter 19: Combining Peptides with Other Approaches

Peptides can do many things, from helping the skin look smoother to guiding the body's signals for growth or repair. However, they rarely work alone in producing major improvements. In most situations, peptides fit best as part of a larger plan. This could include lifestyle habits, other medical treatments, supplements, or even certain therapies. By blending peptides with complementary methods, people might see more stable results and avoid some drawbacks. This chapter explores how peptides can be combined with various approaches, outlining practical ideas and cautions.

---

1. Why Peptides Often Need Support

Peptides are powerful messengers, but the human body is intricate. Changing one signal often depends on other signals, resources, and environmental factors. For example, a peptide that prompts muscle repair will be less effective if a person lacks enough protein in their diet to build new muscle tissue. A peptide that supports collagen can only do so much if the skin is damaged daily by intense sun exposure or if the person smokes heavily, which reduces skin health.

Many medical experts say that peptides alone cannot overcome deep-set problems like chronic inflammation or severe metabolic imbalances. They can help manage aspects of these conditions, but real change often requires overall health strategies. In some cases, peptides are like a spark that starts a reaction, but the environment must be right for the reaction to continue.

---

2. Integrating Peptides with Healthy Eating

Eating patterns can significantly influence how well peptides work. Consider a person aiming to lose weight with a peptide that manages appetite or helps regulate blood sugar. If they keep eating lots of sugar or empty-calorie foods, the peptide's effect might be overshadowed. By adding more fiber, protein, and nutrient-rich meals, the appetite signals might work better. They stay fuller for longer, stable blood sugar remains within reach, and the body's signals align.

Similarly, those using collagen or skin-related peptides might benefit from foods rich in vitamins A, C, and E, along with minerals like zinc. These nutrients support skin regeneration. Some experts also suggest drinking enough water to keep tissues hydrated, so peptides can do their job more effectively. In short, pairing peptides with a diet that matches the body's needs can make a noticeable difference.

---

3. Exercise and Physical Activity

Many peptides relate to muscle function, endurance, or weight management. Exercise provides the stimulus that tells the body to adapt. If a person uses a peptide meant to aid muscle growth but never exercises, the muscle signals may be underutilized. Doing even moderate workouts—like resistance training or bodyweight exercises—can amplify the effect of peptides that help with repair or growth. The peptides help speed recovery, and the muscle-building signals from exercise improve their outcome.

In weight control, combining a peptide that helps appetite or metabolism with daily walks, swimming, or cycling can lead to more steady fat loss. The body becomes more responsive to insulin or other signals. People who enjoy sports might also see that a recovery-supporting peptide works better if they have a balanced training plan, rest enough between sessions, and eat enough protein. Without these basic steps, the peptide's benefits can be small.

---

4. Peptides and Sleep Habits

Sleep is when the body does much of its repair and reset. Growth hormone—often linked to peptide therapies—peaks during deep sleep. If a person is taking a peptide that either boosts or mimics growth signals, poor sleep might sabotage the outcome. They lose that vital window where tissues regenerate. Getting 7 to 9 hours of quality rest can stabilize hormones, reduce stress, and allow peptides to work under optimal conditions.

Furthermore, some peptides influence sleep-wake cycles or stress responses directly. If those are used without healthy sleep habits, results may be inconsistent. Experts on sleep medicine often say that no supplement can fully fix problems caused by chronic sleep deprivation. Instead, combining peptides with good sleep hygiene—like a consistent bedtime, reduced screen time at night, and a cool, dark room—offers a more solid chance of seeing benefits.

---

5. Mixing Peptides with Medical Treatments

People with serious health issues might combine peptides with prescribed drugs or therapies. A few scenarios:

1. **Diabetes Management**: A patient taking a peptide that helps insulin release may still rely on insulin injections or oral medications. Adjusting doses safely requires doctor supervision so that blood sugar does not drop too low.
2. **Autoimmune Disorders**: If someone is on immunosuppressant drugs, a peptide that calms inflammation could help, but it must be balanced so the immune system is not overly weakened.
3. **Joint or Bone Health**: A person with arthritis might add a collagen-boosting peptide to standard anti-inflammatory treatments, plus physical therapy, to help reduce pain and improve mobility.

In each case, the doctor monitors for interactions or overlapping side effects. It might be necessary to shift dosages of existing medications as the peptide changes the body's responses. Medical staff should know which peptides someone is using, even if they are over-the-counter, so they can advise on safe and effective combinations.

---

6. Supplements That May Complement Peptides

Beyond basic nutrition, people often use vitamins, minerals, herbs, or other supplements. Some of these can enhance what peptides do, while others might conflict. For instance:

- **Protein Powders**: If a peptide supports muscle repair, extra protein intake can give raw materials for building muscle.
- **Antioxidants**: Certain peptides help reduce inflammation or support skin structure. Adding antioxidants like vitamin C, E, or specific plant extracts might protect cells from damage, enabling the peptide's effects to last.
- **Co-Factors**: Some processes in the body require minerals (zinc, magnesium) or vitamins (B-complex) to function properly. If the peptide influences those processes, a shortage of co-factors might limit progress.

However, mixing too many supplements can be confusing, leading to unexpected interactions. People sometimes assume that more is always better. In reality, synergy requires understanding. For example, a supplement that strongly affects blood pressure could combine poorly with a peptide that also influences blood vessel function. Checking with a healthcare provider or a knowledgeable nutritionist is wise before stacking multiple items.

---

7. Mind-Body Approaches

Stress can undermine peptide-based therapies, whether the peptides are for weight, skin, or anything else. Chronic stress releases hormones like cortisol, which may conflict with beneficial signals. That is why some doctors suggest mind-body practices to maintain balance. Techniques like:

- **Yoga**
- **Breathing Exercises**
- **Meditation**
- **Progressive Muscle Relaxation**

These can lower overall stress and help the body keep stable hormone levels. If someone is using peptides for anxiety or mental health, combining them with therapy sessions (cognitive-behavioral therapy, for instance) or relaxation strategies might bring better, longer-lasting benefits. Peptides might stabilize certain signals in the brain, but addressing thought patterns or stress triggers is still important.

---

8. Improving Skin Outcomes with Layered Care

Skin-oriented peptides, such as those in creams or serums, often work better if the person also protects their skin from damaging factors. For instance:

1. **Sunscreen**: UV light breaks down collagen. A peptide product that encourages collagen might not help much if the skin keeps getting damaged by the sun. Daily sunscreen use helps keep new collagen safer.
2. **Gentle Cleansing**: Harsh soaps or scrubs can strip skin, while peptides need a healthy barrier to be effective.
3. **Hydration**: Drinking water and using moisturizers can help peptides stay active in the skin's layers.
4. **Balanced Diet**: Vitamins and minerals from the inside support the results that peptides bring from the outside.

Adding treatments like chemical peels or microdermabrasion might help some peptides penetrate more deeply, but only if done carefully, according to a dermatologist's guidance. Overdoing exfoliation can inflame the skin, negating any peptide advantages. A layered approach—peptide serum, sun protection, mild exfoliation, consistent moisture—often yields better outcomes than using a peptide product alone.

---

9. Tuning Peptide Use for Athletes

For those who train or compete in sports (while staying within legal rules and not using banned peptides), synergy with a proper training schedule is essential. Overtraining or ignoring rest days can lead to injuries that peptides cannot magically fix. Meanwhile, correct pacing of workouts, enough rest, and suitable nutrition can allow the body to maximize peptides that boost muscle or support recovery.

An athlete might also do physiotherapy or sports massages to reduce tension, or might use compression garments to improve circulation. When these methods are combined with safe peptides that are not on banned lists, the result could be more efficient muscle repair or less soreness. However, the user must be clear on doping regulations, since many performance-enhancing peptides remain off-limits in official sports.

10. Considering Hormone Balance

Peptides can modify how the body uses hormones, such as growth hormone or insulin. If a person already has an imbalance—too little thyroid hormone, for instance—this might reduce the peptide's ability to bring changes in metabolism. Checking general hormone levels can be beneficial if the goal is to address issues like fatigue, weight gain, or slow muscle growth.

A holistic plan could involve:

- **Correcting any hormonal deficiencies** (through medication or diet)
- **Using a peptide that supports metabolic or muscle-related signals**
- **Adjusting everyday habits (sleep, exercise) to stabilize hormones**

Similarly, if a peptide is used without checking broader hormone status, unexpected side effects might appear. A balanced approach means seeing how each factor fits together. For example, if someone with high cortisol (stress hormone) tries a muscle-building peptide, results might be disappointing until the stress levels come down.

11. Medical Supervision for Complex Cases

Complex situations arise when a person has multiple conditions, such as diabetes plus heart disease plus arthritis. They might benefit from different peptides—one for sugar control, another for joint pain—alongside standard drugs. But layering them all at once can be risky. Medical supervision is key, since the combined effects could strain the body in unforeseen ways.

A doctor might phase in peptides gradually, monitoring labs or vital signs to ensure safety. They may also reduce certain medications if the peptide shows success, preventing over-medication. Communication between specialists is crucial: an endocrinologist, a cardiologist, and a rheumatologist might all need to coordinate if multiple health issues intersect. The goal is a stable synergy rather than random piling of therapies.

12. Combining Peptides in Research

Some labs test combos of peptides. One approach is using two or three short chains that each target different cell receptors involved in a disease. This multi-peptide method might prove more effective than a single chain because it tackles multiple angles. For instance, if one peptide reduces inflammation while another stimulates tissue repair, both might be needed for a strong healing response.

However, multi-peptide research is more complex and expensive. Each additional peptide adds a layer of variables. Scientists must confirm no negative interactions or that the peptides do not degrade each other. Still, the concept of synergy is appealing. Future drug cocktails might mix peptides with small-molecule drugs or even gene therapies, forming comprehensive treatment strategies.

---

13. Lifestyle Shifts for Sustainable Results

People often want quick outcomes from a peptide, whether for weight loss, muscle growth, or improved skin. Yet results can fade if underlying habits do not change. A person might gain a healthier shape with an appetite-regulating peptide but regain weight if they drop the peptide and go back to unhealthy eating. Sustainable progress calls for adopting new lifestyle behaviors that stick long-term.

That might include:

- **Meal planning**: Setting consistent times and portion sizes.
- **Regular exercise**: Finding activities they actually enjoy so they will continue over time.
- **Stress reduction**: Practicing relaxation or mindfulness daily.
- **Healthy social support**: Encouraging friends, family, or group classes to stay on track.

Peptides can jump-start improvements, but healthy living cements them. A continuous cycle of using peptides as a "quick fix" can be expensive and frustrating if root issues remain. By weaving peptides into an overall life plan, changes can last beyond the active use of those substances.

14. Avoiding Conflicts Between Different Peptides

Not all peptides go together. Some might vie for the same receptors, or produce opposite signals. For instance, a peptide that slows metabolism and another that speeds it up could send conflicting messages. Or two peptides might rely on the same breakdown pathway in the liver, causing unpredictable levels in the blood. That is why layering multiple peptides should be done carefully, usually under the advice of a knowledgeable professional.

In beauty products, mixing several peptide serums can be wasteful if their pH levels clash or if the formulas neutralize each other. Skincare experts often suggest layering products in a certain order—lighter, water-based formulas first, heavier creams last. If all are applied at once without guidance, peptides might not penetrate properly, or they might degrade. So while synergy is a goal, random mixing can be counterproductive.

---

15. Mindful Expectations

Combining peptides with other methods can raise the chance of success, but each person should maintain realistic expectations. Even with a perfect blend of diet, exercise, and peptide therapy, transformations do not happen overnight. For example, skin rejuvenation might show steady but modest gains over months. Weight management is a slow process; losing or gaining more than a safe range weekly often leads to relapses.

Mindfulness about time frames and potential plateaus helps people stay motivated. If improvements come gradually, they are often more sustainable. Rushing or raising peptide doses to force quick changes might risk side effects. Good results typically follow a consistent, balanced plan. That is why professionals stress setting realistic goals, tracking progress, and adjusting as needed.

---

16. Working with Coaches or Counselors

In some fields, like sports or wellness, people hire coaches or counselors to guide them. A coach familiar with peptides might help design an overall routine that includes training schedules, meal plans, and safe supplementation. A counselor or therapist could assist individuals using peptides for mental health, ensuring they also learn coping strategies or address emotional stressors.

These professionals can help interpret signals—if someone feels more tired after starting a new peptide, is that normal adjustment or an issue to fix? Coaches and counselors can also keep motivation high and ensure the person uses peptides responsibly, not veering into overuse or shady products. This support network makes synergy smoother, as each piece—peptide, habit, mental approach—fits together.

17. Synergy in Specific Populations

Not everyone has the same baseline health. Some groups need special care:

- **Older Adults**: They might benefit from peptides for bone strength or muscle mass, but age-related changes in metabolism or organ function can alter the results. A plan including gentle exercise and nutrient-dense meals might improve peptide outcomes.
- **Teens**: If peptides are used at all, they should be medically supervised. Combining them with healthy puberty or growth patterns can be tricky. Lifestyle guidance is crucial for balanced development.
- **People with Chronic Conditions**: A custom blend of medication, therapy, and peptides can help manage symptoms without overwhelming the body. Frequent medical checkups reduce risks.
- **Women Before/After Pregnancy**: Some peptides might not be safe in pregnancy or nursing. If used postpartum for recovery, they should be part of a broader postpartum plan addressing sleep, nutrition, and mental health.

In each case, synergy means tailoring the approach to the individual's stage of life and medical background.

18. Data Tracking for Better Results

Technology allows people to monitor progress. Someone using a peptide for weight management could track their calorie intake, steps, sleep quality, and daily mood using apps or wearable devices. By correlating these data points with peptide administration, patterns emerge. This can reveal if the peptide works best after a certain meal type or if certain exercises boost its effect.

Doctors or coaches might review these logs, spotting plateaus early and adjusting plans. The same idea applies for skin changes—measuring hydration levels, or taking photos under consistent lighting can show if a peptide-based cream truly helps. Data-driven synergy is more precise than guessing. It also keeps a person motivated by providing evidence of small improvements over time.

---

19. Adjusting Over the Long Term

Peptide needs and responses can shift as a person's goals or health status changes. For instance, after reaching a certain fitness level, the same dose of a muscle peptide might not be necessary. Or if a skin condition resolves, the user might switch to a milder maintenance peptide or a simpler skincare routine. This continuous adaptation is part of synergy—ensuring that everything remains aligned with the current situation.

Staying flexible is important. Holding onto a peptide regimen that was suitable last year might not be correct this year. A person's schedule, environment, or stress level can also change. Therefore, synergy is not a one-time fix but an ongoing process, where you check how your body responds and shift your plan as needed. This approach maximizes benefits and reduces unwanted side effects or wasted resources.

---

20. Conclusion: Making the Most of Peptides Through Integration

Peptides have notable promise, but they do not work in a vacuum. Real progress happens when they are combined thoughtfully with good nutrition, exercise, medical treatments, or daily habits that create a supportive environment. The synergy principle applies across fields—from athletes trying to reach peak performance, to older adults seeking gentle improvements, to those managing chronic conditions, or even people wanting healthier-looking skin.

By blending peptides with proven methods, individuals can often see more lasting and profound results than if they used peptides alone. This requires being open to guidance, staying aware of interactions, and taking ownership of one's overall health. Peptides can amplify the effects of positive changes, but they rely on the foundation those changes provide. Whether it is balancing hormones, boosting collagen, or tuning the immune system, a plan that looks at the bigger picture is key. Peptides become valuable partners, rather than isolated solutions, in the quest for better health and well-being.

Chapter 20: Creating a Personal Peptide Plan

Peptides can support different goals, such as healthier skin, balanced weight, better muscle repair, or specific wellness targets. But using peptides well often means having a plan. If you are thinking about introducing peptides into your life, it helps to know how to do so in a thoughtful way rather than trying random products with no direction. This chapter is about forming a personal peptide plan that fits your own needs, body, and lifestyle. By following a structured approach, you can reduce guesswork, avoid wasted effort, and raise your chances of safe, consistent results.

Below, we will look at how to gather the right information, define goals, pick the best peptide choices, decide on dosages or product formats, watch for progress, and adjust as you go. We will also cover practical issues, such as finding reliable sources, deciding whether to seek medical help, and mixing peptides with your everyday habits in a balanced way. While each person's plan will vary, the steps described here can serve as a framework to adapt to your own case.

---

1. Clarify Your Reasons for Using Peptides

The first step is to be very clear about why you want to use peptides. Different goals call for different types of peptides, time frames, or ways to apply them. Maybe you want:

- **Improved Skin Appearance**: Reducing fine lines, boosting firmness, or brightening.
- **Weight Support**: Helping with appetite signals, supporting metabolism, or managing energy levels.
- **Muscle Repair or Growth**: Speeding recovery after workouts, supporting muscle maintenance in later adulthood, or addressing specific muscle concerns.
- **Extra Help in Overall Wellness**: A mild lift for issues like tiredness, slow hair growth, or minor concerns with hormone balance.

Some people have multiple goals, which can add complexity. In that case, it is best to rank them: which is most important, and which can wait or be handled later? Trying to fix too many things at once can lead to confusion. By focusing on the most critical targets first, you can pick peptides that match those priorities. Over time, you might add or change peptides if you meet your first aims or if new needs appear.

2. Gather Basic Information About Your Health

Peptide effects depend partly on your overall condition. If you rarely see a doctor or do not have recent health data, it might help to do a simple checkup. Even if you feel healthy, basic measurements such as blood pressure, blood sugar, and body composition can be useful. Having that info can serve as a baseline before starting a peptide plan. If you have concerns about hormones, digestion, or immune issues, you might also consider more specific tests. These could include thyroid function, vitamin levels, or a basic hormone panel.

This step is optional if you are only planning mild, over-the-counter peptide products. But if you aim to address bigger issues—like major weight management or muscle therapy—it is best to have some medical context. You do not want to rely on guesswork if an underlying condition could affect how your body responds. Plus, if you plan to use prescription peptides, a doctor will likely require these details anyway.

3. Choose the Right Peptide or Product

Once you know your main goal and have a sense of your health baseline, it is time to pick which peptide or product makes sense. The choices can be confusing because many brands use the word "peptide" without clarifying details. Here are some tips:

1. **Check the Specific Name**: If you see "contains peptides," that is vague. A better label might say something like "Argireline (Acetyl Hexapeptide-8) cream" or "Palmitoyl Tripeptide-1 serum."
2. **Look for Studies or Evidence**: Many cosmetic peptides have small studies showing they help with certain skin aspects. If you want deeper results, see if the brand offers any references. For medical peptides (like those for blood sugar), look for official approvals or recognized research.
3. **Consider Format**: Topical peptides (creams, serums) often target local areas like skin. Oral supplements might be best for collagen or general

wellness peptides, though absorption can be uncertain. Injections give more direct action but usually require a prescription or medical supervision.
4. **Ask a Professional**: If you are unsure, a dermatologist, endocrinologist, or knowledgeable health practitioner can guide you to the safest and most effective options.

It is also wise to start simple rather than layering many peptides at once. For example, if your main need is smoother skin, pick a well-known peptide product. Use it consistently for at least a month to see how you respond. If you mix multiple new items, you will not know which one is truly helping or if any are causing side effects.

---

4. Decide How to Incorporate Peptides into Your Routine

Any plan needs a practical schedule. Many peptides work better with consistent use. If it is a cream, will you apply it each morning or before bed? If it is an oral supplement, do you take it with meals or on an empty stomach? If it is an injection, do you have the skills to self-inject, or will you visit a clinic?

Writing down these details can prevent confusion. For example, if you take a peptide that regulates appetite, you might time it a short while before your main meal, so you do not overeat. If you have a muscle-peptide injection, maybe you do it post-workout, when your muscles are primed for repair.

Consider day-to-day life. If you travel often, how will you store a peptide that needs refrigeration? If you have a busy morning, can you switch a topical product to nighttime to ensure you do not skip it? The plan should fit your lifestyle, or you may forget or find it too much trouble, which ruins consistency.

---

5. Set Realistic Goals and Timelines

Peptides, like most health interventions, take time to show effects. The body's cells need to use the signals sent by these molecules. Whether you are aiming to reduce wrinkles, drop a few pounds, or gain muscle tone, do not expect instant changes. Set a timeline that gives your body a fair chance to respond. This might be:

- **Skin Improvements**: At least 4–8 weeks to notice small changes in smoothness or firmness.
- **Weight Shifts**: If using an appetite-related peptide, you may see early changes in cravings, but actual weight loss can take many weeks. A safe rate is often around 1–2 pounds lost per week, not huge drops overnight.
- **Muscle Gains or Recovery**: You might see a difference in soreness within days, but actual muscle growth may take a month or more, especially if combined with workouts.

By outlining these timelines, you manage your own hopes. Otherwise, you risk quitting early because you think "it doesn't work," when in fact you just needed more patience. It also helps to define specific markers of success. For example, with weight management, you could track waist circumference or body composition, not just scale weight, to get a broader view of your progress.

6. Combine Peptide Use with Supportive Habits

Think of peptides as part of a bigger puzzle. The other pieces might include a balanced eating pattern, consistent exercise, solid sleep, and stress management. If you have done a previous chapter's reading on synergy, you know that small changes in each area can add up. When you line up your habits with your peptide choice, you create an environment that helps the peptide do its best work.

Possible supportive steps:

- **Skin Plan**: Peptide serum + daily sunscreen + gentle cleansing + healthy fats in your diet.
- **Weight Plan**: Appetite peptide + a meal schedule + moderate exercise + watching overall calorie balance.
- **Muscle Plan**: Repair peptide + protein-rich meals + a mix of resistance workouts + enough rest days.
- **General Wellness**: Mild supportive peptide + basic vitamins (if needed) + stress reduction + consistent bedtime routine.

Make changes slowly if it feels overwhelming. Add or adjust one habit at a time, so it becomes part of your normal routine. If you try a huge overhaul instantly, it can be hard to track which things are helping and which are not. You may also lose motivation if you attempt too many drastic changes.

7. Watch for Possible Side Effects or Interactions

Even when used carefully, peptides can have drawbacks or interactions. Keep an eye out for any unusual signs after you start. Common mild issues can include:

- **Topical Irritation**: Redness, itching, or dryness where a cream is applied.
- **Digestive Upset**: If you are taking oral peptides, you might notice bloating, minor cramps, or changes in bowel habits.
- **Energy Shifts**: Some peptides might alter your energy levels or sleep patterns, especially in the first few days.
- **Changes in Blood Pressure or Heart Rate**: More likely with certain peptides that affect metabolism or blood vessel function.

If side effects are mild and fade quickly, you can continue while keeping notes. If they are more intense or last longer, reduce the dosage, skip the product for a day to see if you feel better, or contact a health professional. It can help to track what time you used the peptide, how you felt after, and any other variables such as new foods or workouts. This record can guide decisions on whether to continue or adjust the plan.

---

8. Keep a Simple Record or Log

One of the best ways to stay organized is by writing down a log. This can be a notebook, an app, or a spreadsheet. You do not need to make it complicated. Basic details:

- **Date and Time**: When you used the peptide or supplement.
- **Dose or Amount**: If it is a cream, note how much you used (perhaps a pea-sized dot). If it is oral, the milligrams or capsules.
- **Any Notable Reactions**: How you felt, energy levels, mood shifts, any skin changes.
- **Progress Markers**: Weekly weight, a monthly tape measure for waist or hips, muscle strength numbers, or skin photos in the same lighting.

This approach helps you see trends. Over a month or two, you might notice that you feel better on days after a good night's sleep. Or you might realize a certain dose works best for you, while going higher causes headaches. Instead of guessing, you have a record that reveals patterns. If you later talk to a doctor or coach, you can show them these notes, giving them a clearer picture of what has happened.

9. Revisit and Adjust the Plan

A personal peptide plan is not fixed in stone. Bodies change, goals shift, and new data might emerge about a product's efficacy. Every few weeks or months, step back and see if you are on track. Ask yourself:

- **Are my original goals still relevant?** Maybe you reached the primary goal already, or your life priorities changed.
- **Is the peptide helping?** If you are not seeing any gains after giving it enough time, maybe you need to switch to another product or brand. Or maybe it is time to add a small second peptide if the first one only addressed part of the issue.
- **Are there any new side effects?** If new concerns pop up, you might have introduced a conflict with other supplements or changed your routine in a way that affects how the peptide works.
- **Do I need a medical opinion?** If the plan is getting more advanced, it might be time to visit a doctor or specialist, especially if you suspect hormone issues or if you want stronger, prescription-level peptides.

By reviewing the plan at set intervals—perhaps every four to six weeks—you can spot when it needs fine-tuning. If everything is going smoothly, you might keep the same approach for a while. If you feel stuck, you could explore the next step or consult a professional for fresh advice.

---

10. Finding Reliable Sources and Products

A major part of any personal plan is ensuring you have a trustworthy product. With the popularity of peptides, there are many questionable sellers. Steps to pick a reliable source:

1. **Check for Quality Marks**: If it is a cosmetic or supplement, look for any independent lab testing or certifications. For prescription peptides, use a licensed pharmacy or clinic.
2. **Avoid Extreme Claims**: If a website promises instant transformations, you might want to dig deeper. Overblown claims often mean the seller is hype-driven.

3. **Look for Clear Ingredient Lists**: Genuine brands often list the exact peptide names. Vague or missing details are suspicious.
4. **Read Reviews Wisely**: Online feedback can be faked, but if a brand has many consistent reviews on different platforms, it may be more trustworthy. Still, approach glowing testimonials with caution, especially if they sound too good to be true.
5. **Check Company Contact Info**: Reputable makers typically have a real address, phone number, or email for customer questions. If contact details are hidden, that is a red flag.

Also, be aware of cost. Peptide production can be expensive, so if you see a product sold at a fraction of the normal price, it might be a counterfeit or watered-down version. That is not always the case, but be cautious. If possible, start with a small order to test quality before committing to a bigger purchase.

---

11. Discussing with Health Experts

Though some peptides are sold over the counter, it can be wise to share your plan with a healthcare provider, especially if you have any ongoing health condition or if you plan to use multiple products. A doctor or a nutrition specialist might spot potential risks or tell you if your plan conflicts with existing medications. They can also track your progress from a medical standpoint, checking if your blood work changes or if certain markers improve.

If you are worried that your doctor might dismiss peptides outright, you can prepare by bringing reputable information or referencing small studies. A thoughtful approach can open a balanced conversation. If your doctor remains opposed, you might seek a second opinion, but do so responsibly. You do not want to ignore valid medical advice.

---

12. Considering Costs and Budget

You should also decide on a budget. Some high-end peptide products, especially prescription ones or advanced cosmetic formulations, can cost quite a bit. Make sure the expense fits your financial situation. If a certain approach is too costly to maintain, look for simpler or more affordable options. Perhaps a single well-formulated product is enough, rather than multiple items. Or consider rotating usage—using a product steadily for a few months, then taking a break if that is safe and supported by the brand's guidance.

If you keep adding more supplements, gym memberships, special foods, or medical consults, the costs can become large. A personal plan that is unsustainable in cost might not last. Better to choose realistic steps that you can handle long-term, which is how many real improvements take hold.

---

13. Handling Changes in Motivation

Motivation can shift over time. In the beginning, you might be excited about starting your peptide plan, but then daily life distractions set in. You might skip some doses or forget to apply that face cream. You might lose track of your meal changes. That is normal. A few strategies can help:

- **Reminders**: Use alarms on your phone or daily checklists. Mark them off when you apply or take the peptide.
- **Habit Linking**: Attach the new habit to a routine you already have. For instance, keep your peptide cream next to your toothbrush, so you remember to use it each morning.
- **Measure Progress**: Seeing even slight improvements can keep you on track. For instance, you might notice your skin feels more supple, or your scale shows a small change in weight.
- **Reward Yourself**: Plan a simple, healthy treat or a relaxing activity when you meet a small milestone, like two weeks of consistent usage.

These points do not guarantee perfect consistency, but they can reduce slip-ups. If you do go off track for a few days, do not feel it is ruined. Just resume your plan as soon as you can. Long-term consistency matters more than minor lapses.

---

14. Planning for Maintenance

Once you reach a milestone—such as a certain skin improvement or weight target—you may wonder if you need to keep using the peptide at the same level.

Often, you can shift to a "maintenance mode." That might mean using a smaller dose, applying a cream less frequently, or cycling on and off the product. Some peptides can be paused without losing all benefits, while others need ongoing use to keep the signals active.

Each product might have guidelines on maintenance. If not, you can experiment carefully, cutting back the frequency in small steps. Watch if changes slip away. If they do, you can return to your old routine or find a middle ground. Maintenance is personal. Some folks like a daily approach, others do fine with every other day. Keep in mind that your body changes with age, environment, and stress. Over the long haul, you might fine-tune the plan multiple times.

---

15. Involving Supportive Partners

It can help to have someone else aware of your plan. Maybe a friend is also interested in peptides, or a partner is curious about your progress. They can offer reminders or encouragement. If you live with someone, tell them about your schedule, so they understand why you are mixing certain supplements or applying certain creams at specific times. This shared understanding can smooth out daily life, reduce misunderstandings, and keep you motivated.

You could also look for online communities focused on the specific peptide use you are interested in. For example, groups discussing collagen for skin, or forums where individuals share tips about appetite-managing peptides. Take these discussions with a healthy dose of caution, though—advice from strangers is not always correct or safe. Still, supportive groups can provide practical suggestions on daily routines or ways to handle side effects. Just double-check any major advice with reliable sources or health professionals.

---

16. Balancing Risks and Benefits

Each person weighs the potential gains against any downsides. For a mild peptide used in a skin cream, the risk is often quite low. For a stronger, prescription-based muscle or hormonal peptide, the stakes might be higher. The key is deciding whether the improvement in well-being, look, or function is worth the financial cost, the effort of consistent use, and the possibility of side effects.

If you sense that you are diving into a complicated or very strong peptide approach just for minor reasons, you might pause and see if simpler methods exist. For instance, if a standard exercise program and better sleep might help your muscle or weight needs without advanced peptides, that might be safer and cheaper. Peptides are best used when they fill a gap that other methods alone cannot handle effectively, or when they speed up or enhance a well-rounded plan.

17. Cultural and Personal Values

People differ in how they feel about changing their body with peptides. Some see it as a modern tool, no different from taking vitamins or following a diet plan. Others worry it is artificial or unnatural. Your personal beliefs should guide how comfortable you are with certain peptides or usage levels. If you feel uneasy about a daily injection to improve minor features, that might clash with your values. If, on the other hand, you are open to science-based solutions, you may see no issue.

It can also depend on local culture. In places where advanced beauty treatments are common, adding a peptide product might seem normal. In other areas, people might be more cautious or view it as unusual. Respecting your own values—and the context around you—helps keep your plan in harmony with your life rather than causing inner conflict.

18. Stepping Up to Prescription Peptides

If your aims go beyond mild everyday issues, you may consider prescription peptides that address deeper concerns. Examples are peptides for serious hormone imbalances or advanced cases of insulin regulation. These are not items you just buy online. They involve a medical process:

1. **Consult a Qualified Doctor**: Explain your situation in detail. Show any records or logs you have maintained.
2. **Undergo Checks**: You might need blood tests or scans to confirm what is causing your symptoms.

3. **Discuss Options**: A prescription peptide might be one of several therapies. The doctor should lay out benefits, risks, and the plan for monitoring.
4. **Agree on a Schedule**: Some prescription peptides require cycles or specific times of day. You might also have check-ins to track your progress.

Prescription peptides can bring bigger effects but also bigger responsibilities. Follow instructions carefully, store them as directed, and keep your checkups. This is particularly relevant for people with conditions like advanced arthritis, complicated metabolic disorders, or serious muscle wasting. The payoff can be significant if used wisely.

---

19. Looking at Long-Term Goals

A personal peptide plan is often one piece of a longer path for health or personal development. For instance, if you want to maintain an active lifestyle into older age, you might rely on certain peptides intermittently while sticking to a routine of safe exercise, balanced nutrition, and regular doctor visits. If your focus is on a certain aesthetic, you might combine periodic skin-peptide products with professional procedures in a clinic, plus a daily skincare regimen at home.

Thinking five or ten years ahead keeps your plan from being just a short fix. Ask yourself: Will I still want to continue these peptides in a year or two? Is there a plan to reduce usage once I reach certain changes? By having a broader view, you avoid short-lived fads. Instead, you fold peptides into your life as tools that can help at certain stages, always balanced with your overall well-being.

---

20. Bringing It All Together

Creating a personal peptide plan is about making smart, informed choices in line with your goals, health profile, and daily habits. The steps can be summarized as follows:

1. **Identify Your Main Goals**: Whether skin, weight, muscle, or general health, be precise.

2. **Know Your Body**: Gather any relevant health checks or input from professionals.
3. **Select a Reliable Peptide or Product**: Look for clarity, evidence, and a trustworthy brand.
4. **Set a Usage Schedule**: Time of day, frequency, method of application or ingestion.
5. **Outline Realistic Timelines**: Expect changes to take weeks or months, not days.
6. **Blend with Supporting Habits**: Nutrition, exercise, stress management, and more.
7. **Track Effects and Adjust**: Keep a log, note side effects, tweak as needed, and do periodic reviews.
8. **Stay Ethical and Safe**: Follow legal or medical guidelines, be honest with providers, and respect your body's signals.

By following these steps, you cut down on guesswork or random tries. You also build a foundation that can carry you forward if you decide to expand your plan later. The best peptide users are those who stay curious, measure progress, and adapt responsibly.

That said, peptides are not magic. They are helpers that support your body's signals. Everything else—your daily routines, self-discipline, environment—plays a big part in whether you see short-lived or lasting improvements. If you take your time and approach it wisely, peptides can become a valuable tool in your toolkit, used in moderation and aligned with your personal goals.

In summary, your personal peptide plan should grow with you. Revisit it whenever something shifts in your health or lifestyle. Keep learning about new data or new peptides if they are relevant, but do not jump on every trend. With consistency, caution, and realistic views, you can use peptides to enhance specific areas of your life while maintaining overall balance. Through careful planning, you will likely get more stable benefits, minimize risks, and feel that your efforts truly fit who you are and what you want in the long run.

www.ingramcontent.com/pod-product-compliance
Lightning Source LLC
LaVergne TN
LVHW012103070526
838202LV00056B/5605